THE
POSTPARTUM
DEPRESSION
WORKBOOK

THE
POSTPARTUM
DEPRESSION
WORKBOOK

Strategies to Overcome
Negative Thoughts, Calm Stress,
and Improve Your Mood

Abigail Burd, LCSW, PMH-C

**ROCKRIDGE
PRESS**

To L and R, for choosing me as your mother

To M, for making us a family

To my parents, on earth and in heaven

CONTENTS

Part 2:
TOOLS AND STRATEGIES 23

Part 3:
POSTPARTUM DEPRESSION IN REAL LIFE 97

REMEMBER, YOU ARE NOT ALONE *143*

INTRODUCTION

One in five women will develop postpartum depression (PPD) after the birth of a baby. Another three or four will just feel like they were hit with a ton of bricks.

I didn't have full-blown PPD, but I was hit hard. I sure wasn't expecting those bricks. I'd worked my entire adult life in the mental health field. I went to graduate school for clinical social work and became licensed. I'd worked in a top university psychiatric training program, learning alongside psychiatry residents. But I'd barely heard of PPD.

When I was pregnant, my OB-GYN took my vitals and screened me each visit for warning signs of preeclampsia. I drank a dreadful sugar drink to rule out gestational diabetes. But *not one* health-care provider warned me about the most common complication of childbirth.

I read every book I could on pregnancy and researched the best car seats, strollers, baby carriers, and diaper systems. Yet as I became a new mom myself, I was shocked at how hard *everything* was.

I was sleep deprived, hormonal, crushed at how little milk I was making, and seriously worried about my baby gaining weight. I was confused by conflicting advice about what to do, and the stakes—my baby's survival—couldn't have been higher.

Fast forward a couple years, as I prepared for my second pregnancy and birth. I did a lot of things differently. To be honest, I had a wonderful experience.

I briefly considered having more and more babies, so I could do it again. Next, I thought I'd train to be a doula, so I could help other birthers. I'd experienced how brutal *and* how transcendental the postpartum stage could be, and how a little bit of support, education, and encouragement could make that difference.

Then, something happened. It was the simplest of things. I was on my second maternity leave, perhaps only a few weeks postpartum. A friend called me. I remember I was at the park, pushing my toddler on the swings, wearing my newborn in a ring sling. The San Diego sun was warm during the October lunch hour.

My friend was anxious. She was overdue with her baby. She wanted to deliver in a birth center but was a day away from being too overdue to be admitted there. We addressed her fears, then looked at what was within her control. I helped her reframe her thoughts and practice things she already knew to bring calm and lift her mood.

And guess what? She had that baby before dinner.

That day I realized I already had the tools to help pregnant and postpartum people. I had been working in a cognitive therapy program and was already skilled at defeating depression and anxiety. Bingo! I just knew I could help clients with postpartum depression.

Ever since then, I have dedicated my therapy practice to helping people with perinatal mood and anxiety disorders. I have been overwhelmed by how powerful evidence-based therapies, such as cognitive behavioral therapy (CBT) and interpersonal psychotherapy (IPT), are at treating and preventing PPD.

I have helped numerous people in my private practice and in my educational programs overcome PPD. I know you can benefit from this material, too.

HOW TO USE THIS BOOK

Welcome! I'm so glad you have decided to prioritize *you* and your mental health.

You are here because you want to feel better. I am hopeful the information and tools here can help you on your journey.

First, a word about you. You might be the biological or gestational parent to your baby, or you might not be. Postpartum depression (PPD) has a hormonal component, and parts of this book refer to birth or pregnancy. However, birth is not a prerequisite for PPD. This book will still be relevant to you if you grew your family through surrogacy, adoption, or other means. Simply skip the parts you don't relate to.

Likewise, you could be among the 1 in 10 partners suffering from a postpartum mood or anxiety disorder. Becoming a parent is a huge transition and has changed your life in potentially drastic ways. Please approach these tools as a resource for you, too.

Last but far from least, if you are a transgestational, genderqueer, or non-binary parent growing your family, you are welcome here. My editors and I questioned the use of gendered language, such as *women* or *mother*. At times, I have used "women" if it was the term used in research (it is in the majority of recent PPD studies). And although we thought terms like *mother, mom,* and *matrescence* were an important concept to use for many in this season of life, I hope they do not diminish your sense of being welcome and visible. Please ignore what is not relevant and substitute the terms that aid you in your transition to parenthood.

Because I know time is in short supply for new parents, I have organized this workbook to be easy to navigate. Although it would be helpful to read and work through the entire workbook, you are encouraged to jump to a specific tool or exercise that speaks to your current concern.

This workbook is divided into three parts.

Part 1: "Understanding Your Postpartum Depression" introduces you to the most common perinatal mood disorder. It covers the common signs of PPD, what it is and isn't, and its most common risk factors. It describes the causes of PPD, provides a quiz to help you determine whether you might have it, discusses how it impacts partners as well as the birth parent, and covers what you can do about it.

Part 2: "Tools and Strategies" takes a deep dive into practical solutions. You will find exercises, worksheets, quizzes, and other interactive tools that are grounded in cognitive behavioral therapy (CBT), a powerful approach shown by research to help you overcome PPD. The exercises will lead you through thoughts, feelings, behaviors, and skills aimed at understanding, coping with, and moving through your PPD symptoms and self-care options.

Part 3: "Postpartum Depression in Real Life" asks and answers the concerns of parents like you. I would never share the private stories of any of my therapy clients. Those I guard as confidential. However, the issues raised in part 3 are ones that *all my clients* ask about. Each of the real-life situations is addressed with relevant advice, simple tips, and additional CBT exercises.

My hope is that you can use this workbook either as a quick fix in the moments you need it most or as a comprehensive toolbox designed to equip you with all the mental health tools you need to navigate the transition to becoming a healthy and happy parent.

Part 1

Understanding Your Postpartum Depression

My guess, if you've bought this book, is that you have heard of postpartum depression (PPD). But how well do you understand it?

As our starting point, let's go over the symptoms of PPD and explore whether they relate to you. You will have a chance to reflect and write as we dive deeper into PPD, covering what it is and isn't, and the most common risk factors. Next, I'll cover the causes of PPD, provide a quiz for you to see if you might have it, and discuss how it impacts both parents. Finally, we'll start to discuss what you can do about it. Spoiler: We can do a lot to make it better.

What Are the Symptoms?

Let's go over the symptoms of PPD. The following checklist cannot replace an actual assessment and diagnosis by a licensed professional, but it can be a place to start. PPD, or major depression with peripartum onset, might be diagnosed if you have five or more of the following symptoms and they have lasted **most of the day, nearly every day, for the past two weeks**. As you read through the list, place a check mark next to each symptom you have experienced.

- ☑ Depressed mood
- ☑ Loss of interest or pleasure in things you normally enjoy
- ☑ Significant changes in appetite and/or weight
- ☐ Difficulty sleeping or sleeping too much
- ☑ Psychomotor agitation (e.g., pacing, fidgeting, tapping hands/legs) or retardation (feeling slowed down physically or mentally)
- ☑ Fatigue or loss of energy
- ☐ Difficulty concentrating or indecisiveness
- ☑ Feelings of worthlessness
- ☑ Excessive or inappropriate guilt
- ☐ Thoughts of death or suicide

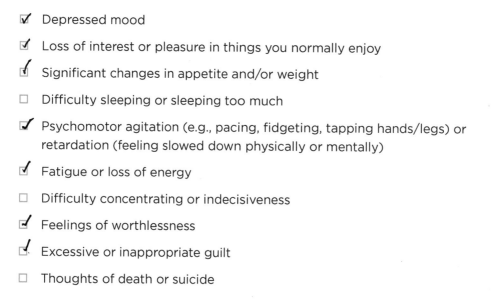

If you have thoughts of harming yourself, your baby, or someone else, please do not be embarrassed, but **do not delay** seeking help immediately. About one in five mothers with PPD has thoughts of harming themselves. It is very important that you reach out! In the United States, the National Suicide Prevention Lifeline is 1-800-273-8255, or you can call 911. The crisis text line is available 24/7 in the United States and Canada (text 741741), the UK (text 85258), and Ireland (text 086 1800 280). International hotlines are listed on SuicideStop.com.

In addition to the above symptoms of depression, sometimes PPD looks different from the depression we might experience during other times in our lives. Some of my clients describe it as an anxious depression. On the other hand, some are surprised to find themselves not sad but full of anger, irritability, and even rage.

In fact, PPD often looks more like anxiety than depression. Many of us in my field now prefer the term *perinatal mood and anxiety disorders*, or PMADs, to cover both anxiety and depression, both during pregnancy and after. (*Perinatal* refers to before pregnancy, during pregnancy, and after birth or a pregnancy loss.) In this workbook, we will use both terms. My hope is that the tools here will help you with the symptoms of both depression and anxiety.

Since PPD doesn't always look like depression, here are some other warning symptoms to look out for. Put a check mark next to each one you have experienced.

- ☑ Do you feel like you just aren't yourself?
- ☑ Are you withdrawing from supportive/helpful people?
- ☑ Do you regret having a baby? Feel like it was a mistake?
- ☑ Are you losing your temper more easily?
- ☑ Are you afraid of losing control?
- ☐ Do you feel like you can't shake off the bad feelings, no matter what you try?
- ☑ Do you tell everyone you are fine, but feel anything but?
- ☑ Are you afraid to tell others how you feel because they won't understand or will think there is something worse wrong with you?
- ☐ Do you feel like your baby would be better off without you?
- ☐ Do you have a lack of interest in your baby?
- ☑ Are you afraid to be alone with your baby?
- ☑ Do you feel like you don't/can't love your baby?
- ☑ Are you fighting more than usual with your partner?
- ☑ Do you have trouble sleeping, even when the baby is asleep?
- ☐ Do any scary or unwanted thoughts come into your mind?
- ☐ Do you have thoughts of running away from your family?
- ☑ Do you feel like a failure as a mother?
- ☑ Have you given up hope that things will get better?

Remember, different people experience PPD in different ways. These are just a few of the symptoms my clients with PMADs have revealed. You don't have to have all of these symptoms. If you have even one, it's worth exploring or discussing with someone else.

However, even if you relate to many of these symptoms, that doesn't give you an automatic diagnosis or label. It's just an indication that you might need a little more support, mama. The fact that you are reading this workbook shows you are already off to a great start. You want to feel better. Maybe you want to be the best *you* possible for your family. Or maybe you're doing it just because *you* want to. You can and you will feel better. You deserve to.

Now that you know about a few of the ways other people feel with PPD or PMADs, think about how you have been feeling. Make a list of the symptoms you have noticed. Then write down comments about the "normal" you, or the you before the baby.

ME NOW:

ME BEFORE:

What Is Postpartum Depression?

Essentially, postpartum depression (PPD) is depression occurring during the first year after giving birth. A well-respected study of 10,000 women published in *JAMA Psychiatry* in 2013 documented that 21 percent had PPD in the first year. For simplicity's sake, we can call this one in five.

But perinatal psychotherapists, like me, find that parents may first seek therapy well past the first year. We still see PPD two, three, or more years later. Why? Sadly, it's usually because parents have struggled for years before finally reaching out for help. (Stop and give yourself a pat on the back for using this workbook now. It takes bravery and courage to take this step.)

Did you know PPD sometimes starts during pregnancy? As I mentioned, therapists like me are starting to favor the term perinatal mood or anxiety disorder, or PMAD. Mood disorders encompass both depressive and bipolar disorders. Anxiety disorders include generalized anxiety, obsessive-compulsive disorder (OCD), and posttraumatic stress.

If you are currently pregnant, trying to conceive, or well past 12 months postpartum and are experiencing some symptoms of depression, this workbook will definitely still be helpful for you. If you are experiencing other PMADs, you *might* also find some of these tools relevant, as well.

What Isn't PPD?

Some symptoms and disorders might look like PPD, but they are actually something else. It's important to know the difference. We'll discuss some of the most common ones here.

The "Baby Blues"

Approximately 80 percent or more of birthers experience a period of the "baby blues." You might feel tearful, sensitive, and tired. However, the baby blues is not as severe as depression. The baby blues often starts around four days postpartum, as your body experiences hormone shifts, but it usually lifts after two weeks postpartum. If you have been feeling down for longer than two weeks, it's not the baby blues anymore.

Postpartum Bipolar Disorder

Postpartum bipolar disorder is sometimes called manic depression and is most concerning because it could lead to postpartum psychosis (see "Postpartum Psychosis" below). Women with preexisting bipolar disorder are usually encouraged by reproductive psychiatrists to stay on their medication (with exceptions such as Depakote or valproic acid) and to have a plan for getting regular sleep. Definitely discuss your particular plan with your own doctor. If someone is not in the reproductive life cycle, bipolar disorder, and even psychosis, are not that alarming. But for a postpartum woman, it should be addressed right away.

Postpartum Psychosis

Postpartum psychosis is a true psychiatric emergency, marked by hallucinations, disorganized thoughts or speech, and/or delusions. If you or someone you love is experiencing these symptoms, please see a doctor **today**. Psychosis is rare, with only 1 or 2 out of 1,000 women developing it during the postpartum stage. Unfortunately, there are serious consequences if untreated. Of those women with postpartum psychosis, 5 percent die by suicide and 4 percent commit infanticide (the killing of an infant). The biggest risk factor for postpartum psychosis is a previous or current episode of bipolar disorder. Postpartum psychosis is also often exacerbated by sleep deprivation. Again, if you or someone you love is having symptoms of psychosis, please seek help today.

Defining "Normal"

The easiest way to explain the difference between normal ups and downs and depressive or bipolar mood swings is with the Mood State Pyramid.

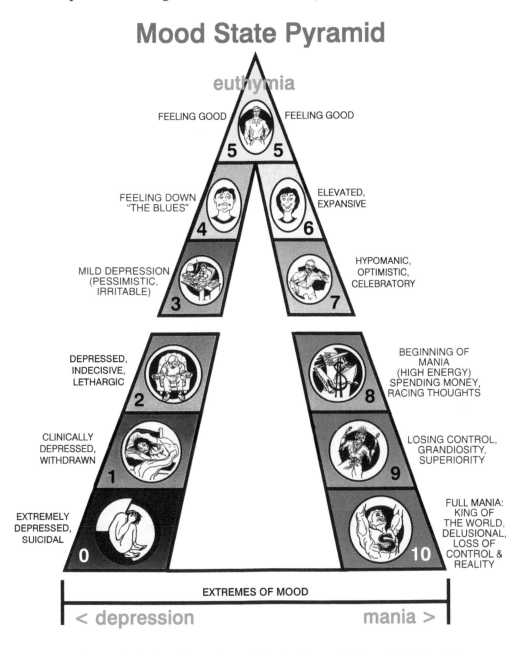

Reprinted with permission from Depression and Bipolar Support Alliance (DBSA) San Diego.

Most people have ups and downs ranging from 3 to 7. This is normal. Clinical depression is represented by the 0 to 2 range. A manic episode is represented by the 8 to 10 range. People suffering from bipolar II disorder experience mood swings ranging from as low as 0 to 2 to as high as 7 or 8. People diagnosed with bipolar I disorder experience true manic episodes, rated 8 or higher.

If your symptoms are better explained by the baby blues, postpartum bipolar disorder, or postpartum psychosis, you might not have PPD.

But what about anxiety? In fact, two-thirds of women with PPD also meet criteria for an anxiety disorder. Yup, you can have both postpartum anxiety and depression at the same time. Let's look more closely at the different forms of anxiety.

Postpartum Anxiety

As mentioned, one in five women has anxiety during pregnancy or in the first year postpartum. I like to think about anxiety as a spectrum. We all experience some anxiety or stress. A little bit can motivate us to do the things we need to do. Too much anxiety gets in the way. If you are having excessive worry about your pregnancy or your baby's health and can't be reassured, think about getting some help. Other concerns are being unable to sleep due to worrying or having panic attacks.

Postpartum Posttraumatic Stress

You might think only veterans can get posttraumatic stress disorder (PTSD). However, any event in which you or someone you love was in serious danger can trigger a posttraumatic response. Approximately 30 percent of births have some kind of trauma, such as the mother's or baby's life being in danger or a stay in the neonatal intensive care unit (NICU). Symptoms of postpartum PTSD include intrusive memories, avoidance of triggers that remind you of what happened, mood changes, difficulty sleeping, and being easily triggered or scared.

Postpartum Obsessive-Compulsive Disorder

Parents suffering with perinatal obsessive-compulsive disorder (OCD) may have obsessions (intrusive, repetitive thoughts) or compulsions (repetitive behaviors driven by a need to reduce anxiety). The most common scary thought experienced with postpartum OCD is a fear that you may deliberately harm your own baby. If you have had this thought and been disturbed by it, please know you are *not alone*. And the fact that this thought bothered you is a great sign that you may have simply had an intrusive thought and are *not* at true risk of infanticide. Other common intrusive worries include fear of contamination, something being wrong with the baby, and accidentally harming the baby. If you have scary thoughts, please do not be afraid to talk about them with someone you trust. The fact that you are worried about hurting your baby most likely means you would never do it and want to protect your infant. But it is very important that you share your fears to break the cycle of secrecy and shame.

Telling the Difference

Bottom line, if you are having any kind of psychosis (including hearing voices, seeing things, or believing things others do not believe) or any thoughts of harming yourself or your baby, *get immediate help* today via emergency services. If you are having any kind of manic symptoms while pregnant or postpartum, please seek an appointment with a psychiatrist *immediately*. On the other hand, if you are having anxiety (including intrusive, scary thoughts or fallout from birth trauma) along with your depression, you are still in the right place.

What Are the Risk Factors for PPD?

PPD does not discriminate. It affects folx from all walks of life. However, some personal characteristics and experiences increase the likelihood of someone developing PPD or another PMAD.

Some people are more at risk than others. Let's see if any of the risk factors apply to you. These factors are known to increase the chances that PPD could impact you. As you read through the list of risks, check off the ones that apply to you.

☐ Previous history of depression

☐ History of physical or sexual abuse, assault, or other trauma

☐ Lack of social support

☐ Either you or your partner were unhappy about the pregnancy

☐ Interpersonal violence

☐ Other issues with your partner

☐ Perfectionism, difficulty asking for help, or both

☐ Traumatic pregnancy or delivery

☐ NICU and/or special needs baby

☐ Multiple births (e.g., twins, etc.)

☐ Financial stress or other life stressors

☐ History of or current drug or alcohol abuse

☐ Distance (physical or emotional) from extended family

☐ Trauma due to racism, marginalization

☐ Family history of perinatal depression or other mental illness

☐ Reproductive loss (miscarriage, stillbirth) and/or infertility

☐ Issues with breastfeeding

☐ Older mom or teen mom

☐ History of premenstrual dysphoric disorder (PMDD) or severe PMS

In addition to the previous list, the following vulnerable populations are at an increased risk of PPD. (This list is by no means exhaustive but should start you thinking.)

Women of color/BIPOC (Black, Indigenous, and people of color). About 20 percent of women develop PPD, but 38 percent of women of color suffer from PPD. Black and Hispanic depressed mothers are more likely to experience multiple adversities and are less likely to receive services than White depressed mothers. Studies show Black and Latinx mothers with PPD are less likely to start treatment, have fewer treatment options, and are less likely to stick with treatment. Indigenous women also have higher rates of perinatal depression. Although all women are now supposed to be screened for depression and anxiety during perinatal visits, a recent study showed racial disparities: Indigenous and multiracial women are less often screened for PPD than White women, Asian women even less, and Black women least often of all.

So Black women are more likely to experience PPD, but even worse, they are three to four times more likely to die from childbirth. Black women who are college educated or over the age of 30 are four to five times more likely to die from pregnancy and birth-related causes than White women. Institutional racism directly and indirectly leads health-care providers to take the concerns of Black women less seriously. The CDC reports that Black women are twice as likely to have their infant die prematurely. Chronic exposure to racism increases physical and mental health problems, as well as rates of miscarriage and infertility. In fact, the lived experience of chronic racism changes the uterus, increasing preeclampsia, negatively impacting the placenta and umbilical cord, and leading to preterm birth and low birth weight. Furthermore, these impacts of lived racism can be seen in birth outcomes a generation later.

Women of color overall have less access to high-quality mental health resources. Although we are finally seeing more awareness around the structural racism impacting pregnant and postpartum parents, much more work is still needed to better support Black mothers. Please see specific resources for Black, Indigenous, and people of color (BIPOC) with PPD on page 147.

LGBTQIA birthing parents. LGBTQIA parents often face heterosexism, cissexism (prejudice or discrimination against people who are transgender, genderqueer, and non-binary), and exclusion from the birth and medical communities. Lesbian women have a higher prevalence of PPD and have increased rates of attempting or considering suicide related to PPD. Bisexual women, as invisible sexual minorities, have an increased risk of PPD if they are currently partnered with a man versus a woman. While more research is needed to document the rate of PPD among transgestational, genderqueer, and non-binary parents, we know they have higher rates of baseline depression, anxiety, and suicide, as well as more experiences of discrimination and trauma.

Single parents. Single mothers are twice as likely as partnered mothers to report depression and anxiety. Even two-parent households are completely overwhelmed with the amount of work to be done. In addition, one major stressor for parents is having adequate childcare they can trust and rely on. Single mothers may feel this stress and guilt all the more.

Intersectionality. Parents who identity with more than one of the above groups may find themselves at an even further disadvantage. For example, a person of color who identifies as a sexual minority may feel ostracized by either group. Even once they have found their "people," they may find fewer of their previous supports are currently in the life stage of becoming parents.

If you are feeling overwhelmed by your number of risk factors, remember you are not alone. You do not need to suffer in silence or feel the burden of being strong and resilient. You are worthy of help and support and deserve to be uplifted.

What Causes PPD?

There are many causes of PPD. Some are biological, and some are psychological, social, or cultural.

Biological factors, especially for birthing parents, include massive hormonal changes, thyroid changes, and the physiological toll of vaginal and surgical births. Other huge hormonal shifts occur when breastfeeding is stopped or reduced or when menstrual cycles return. For all parents, chronic sleep deprivation impacts mood, irritability level, and resilience.

The process of becoming a mother is an intense life transition psychologically. Some compare it to the developmental stage of adolescence and call it *matrescence*, or the "birth of a mother." For some, the birth itself was traumatic, and either your life or the baby's life may have been in serious danger. For others, the birth or breastfeeding experience may be a trigger for past sexual or physical abuse. In addition, you may be experiencing changes in how you view and judge yourself and your performance as a mother.

I often wonder how much PPD we would have if new families had appropriate social support. In modern Western culture, nuclear families are isolated in their individual homes. This is the worst possible setup for new parents. Many traditional societies practice nurturing new parents for 40 days, 6 weeks, 2 months, or a similar amount of time. (You may hear people call this "the fourth trimester.")

When extended family and the community support the new parents, the parents are free to bond with and care for their newborn. In an ideal world, both parents would not have to work or leave the home for other responsibilities. If that is not realistic for you, know that you have a lot of company. Start brainstorming the next best thing. How can you mobilize a support network?

(See "Asking for Help Is Hard" on page 100 to explore this topic further.)

QUIZ: DO I HAVE PPD?

The following quiz comes from the Edinburgh Postnatal Depression Scale, the most widely used screening tool for PPD. Please keep in mind that your score here cannot replace an evaluation by a therapist or doctor and *is not a formal diagnosis*. That said, taking this quiz can give you a good idea of where you fall in the PPD range and if you should seek treatment.

For each statement, mark an X in the box next to the answer that comes closest to how you have felt **over the past seven days**—not just how you feel today.

Over the past seven days:

1. I have been able to laugh and see the funny side of things.

    0 _____ As much as I always could

    1 _____ Not quite so much now

    2 _____ Definitely not so much now

    3 _____ Not at all

2. I have looked forward with enjoyment to things.

    0 _____ As much as I ever did

    1 _____ Rather less than I used to

    2 _____ Definitely less than I used to

    3 _____ Hardly at all

3. I have blamed myself unnecessarily when things went wrong.

    3 _____ Yes, most of the time

    2 _____ Yes, some of the time

    1 _____ Not very often

    0 _____ No, never

4. I have been anxious or worried for no good reason.

    0 _____ No, not at all

    1 _____ Hardly ever

    2 _____ Yes, sometimes

    3 _____ Yes, very often

5. I have felt scared or panicky for no very good reason.

    3 _____ Yes, quite a lot

    2 _____ Yes, sometimes

    1 _____ No, not much

    0 _____ No, not at all

6. Things have been getting on top of me.

    3 _____ Yes, most of the time I haven't been able to cope

    2 _____ Yes, sometimes I haven't been coping as well as usual

    1 _____ No, most of the time I have coped quite well

    0 _____ No, I have been coping as well as ever

7. I have been so unhappy that I have had difficulty sleeping.

    3 _____ Yes, most of the time

    2 _____ Yes, sometimes

    1 _____ Not very often

    0 _____ No, not at all

8. I have felt sad or miserable.

    3 _____ Yes, most of the time

    2 _____ Yes, quite often

    1 _____ Not very often

    0 _____ No, not at all

9. I have been so unhappy that I have been crying.

    3 _____ Yes, most of the time

    2 _____ Yes, quite often

    1 _____ Only occasionally

    0 _____ No, never

10. The thought of harming myself has occurred to me.

    3 _____ Yes, quite often

    2 _____ Sometimes

    1 _____ Hardly ever

    0 _____ Never

Questions from Cox, J. L., Holden, J. M., & Sagovsky, R., "Detection of Postnatal Depression: Development of the 10-Item Edinburgh Postnatal Depression Scale," British Journal of Psychiatry *150 (1987): 782–786. Reprinted with permission.*

SCORING YOUR QUIZ ANSWERS

First, if you marked anything other than 0 on question 10, I would like you to talk with a therapist or doctor. Please talk to someone **today** if you marked a 3. See the suicide prevention resources on page 146.

Now add up the numbers next to your check marks.

My score is _____

Research cautions that some people (depending on culture, gender, and the individual) are more likely to downplay their symptoms. So, even if your score is fairly low, I would still recommend using the tools in this workbook. Please consider therapy at any score as a way to increase your support and feel heard. You may especially want to consider therapy at a score of 10 or above. If you score high, I encourage you to add more treatment than this workbook alone provides. Remember, a workbook cannot replace treatment with someone who can see and hear you.

What Can I Do About My PPD?

Fortunately, PPD is very treatable. Therapy, social support, support groups, medication, nutrition and exercise, and complementary/integrative health can all help.

If you meet with a perinatal psychotherapist, they should help you connect with the right postpartum supports, like the ones above, as well as use an evidence-based therapy to treat PPD. Two forms of therapy or counseling have been shown by research to both treat and prevent PPD: cognitive behavioral therapy (CBT) and interpersonal psychotherapy (IPT). While I will throw a few elements from IPT into this workbook, true IPT is more dependent on the relationship between the therapist and client. Here, I will predominantly draw upon CBT, as exercises from CBT work well both in therapy and in this format.

Indeed, CBT has been shown to reduce PPD symptoms (as measured by the Edinburgh Postnatal Depression Scale, the same quiz as in the last section) when used outside of traditional therapy, including in-home, online, app, and telephone formats. This workbook is not intended to replace therapy, but it is something you could use together with your work with your therapist.

Key features of CBT include:

→ **Goal Oriented.** With CBT, you and your therapist have a clear goal (such as reducing the symptoms of PPD). When CBT is used in an in-home or online format, there is also a clear purpose. Simple talk therapy, on the other hand, is more open and loose.

→ **Time Limited.** Old-school psychodynamic psychotherapy and psychoanalysis can go on for years, the latter with multiple appointments each week. CBT and other time-limited therapies are designed to be completed in 5 to 20 sessions. It is more common to meet once a week or once every two weeks.

→ **Focuses on the Present.** While a CBT therapist may ask about your past to help understand your view of the world and how your past impacts you now, the treatment focuses on the here and now.

CBT works by helping you identify your automatic thoughts, notice how they shape your beliefs, and learn how beliefs lead to emotional and behavioral consequences. For example, have you ever had a thought similar to this: "My partner said something mean/dumb/insensitive, and it made me feel sad/angry"? When something happens or someone says something, it doesn't actually make us feel a certain way. It was simply the activating event (the thing that triggered something else). It is actually our beliefs about what happened, ourselves, and the world that color, or influence, how we then feel.

The chain can be expressed like this: Activating events (A) *lead to* certain Beliefs (B) *that cause* emotional and/or behavioral Consequences (C). You can think of this chain as the ABCs of CBT.

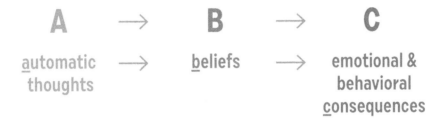

HOW CAN I FIND A THERAPIST WHO SPECIALIZES IN PPD?

Postpartum Support International has made it easier to know if a therapist has training and experience in treating perinatal mood and anxiety disorders. The organization launched a certification in perinatal mental health in 2018. Only providers who meet its standards of training and experience and pass a certification exam can use the initials PMH-C after their name. You can also use its directory, PSIDirectory.com, to search for a specialist worldwide. Search features include filtering based on your health insurance and preferred treatment orientation (such as CBT).

What About Medication?

Here's a myth I bet you've heard before: You can't take medication if you are pregnant or breastfeeding. It's usually followed by a statement like, "You just don't know what effect medication will have on the baby!" Did you know that SSRIs, the most common class of antidepressants, are in fact the most studied medication in pregnancy?

There are many myths about meds, even within the medical community, so consider a second opinion from a reproductive psychiatrist if your OB-GYN—or sister, hairdresser, or social media friend—tells you to stop taking them. Many OB-GYNs have never been trained in psychiatry and many psychiatrists have never been trained in pregnancy or lactation. This double gap in knowledge highlights the need for expert advice from reproductive psychiatrists. There might not be one in your area, but you can have your doctor call the PSI Perinatal Psychiatric Consult Line at 1-800-944-4773, extension 4.

See the sections "To Medicate or Not to Medicate" on page 73 and "Pros and Cons of Medication" on page 79 for more information.

Regardless of whether you ultimately decide that medication is right for you, therapy can be helpful for any severity of PPD.

What Are the Risks of *Not* Treating PPD?

When faced with the decision to act or not to act, you can be predisposed to inaction by the lethargy and indecisiveness caused by PPD. Some parents, and particularly female-identified parents, are willing to suffer if they think they are doing the best thing for their child.

Please understand that treating your PPD is the best thing you can do for your baby.

Untreated or undertreated depression has lasting consequences during pregnancy, in the postpartum stage, and when parenting.

A pregnant woman's untreated depression is dangerous to her unborn baby's health. Some of the other risks of untreated depression during pregnancy are miscarriage, preeclampsia, and reduced fetal responsiveness in utero.

Children born to depressed mothers are more likely to have delayed development and reduced attachment and behavioral problems throughout childhood and into adolescence. Untreated PMADs in either parent have negative effects on the infant–caregiver relationship. As a result, untreated PMADs affect early developmental outcomes of infants, including neurological and regulatory development, and developmental milestones. The most dangerous outcomes of untreated perinatal mental illness are suicide or infanticide.

There is also a massive financial cost to untreated PMADs. One study, published at the time of this writing, used a cost-of-illness model to estimate the cost of untreated PMADs at $14 billion in the United States alone. The average cost per mother and baby was $31,800.

If you are worried about lasting effects on your child, one of the best things you can do for your baby is to keep working on your PPD symptoms. Although depression can lower your ability to respond appropriately to your baby's needs, research indicates CBT helps to correct that. Parents who use CBT to manage their depression are able to catch up and bond better with their baby.

If you were on the fence about doing something about your perinatal depression or anxiety, please consider taking action now. It will be better for your child, and *you* deserve to feel better, too.

You're Not Alone

Roughly 3.8 million Americans gave birth last year. From that we can extrapolate that about 760,000 are currently suffering from PPD, using current statistics. Worldwide, when 140 million give birth annually, 28 million may be suffering from PPD. That's 28 *million* right now (not to mention 14 million partners). Clearly, you are not alone.

You may feel lonely, however. PPD is the most underdiagnosed complication of childbirth. Doctors and others are finally getting better at screening for PPD. Not until 2016 did the United States Preventive Services Task Force and the American College of Obstetricians and Gynecologists recommend routinely screening pregnant and postpartum women for depression.

Despite increased awareness and screening, many are still afraid to speak up. Why?

Stigma is the fear of judgment. We may be afraid others will think we are to blame or that we're bad mothers if we voice anything less than maternal bliss.

But you know what? Caring mothers get help. The symptoms of PPD are real—they are not in your head. (If anything, they are in your body and nervous system.) And, fortunately, PPD is very treatable. Many people find their symptoms are only temporary, but dealing with them does take some work. Are you willing to start?

Did you know dads and non-birthing partners can also suffer from PPD?

One in 10 new fathers meets the criteria for paternal perinatal depression. The biggest risk factor is if the mom has PPD. In men, PPD might look different. Rather than sadness, look out for irritability, anger, and an increase in escaping behaviors like video games and substance abuse. Men also experience hormonal shifts. Lower testosterone levels, thought to improve bonding and gentleness after the birth of a baby, are also associated with increased PPD in fathers.

As there is an increased prevalence of depression in the LGBTQIA community, it comes as no surprise that female, non-binary, and trans partners are at an even higher risk of developing PPD. Being the gestational carrier is not a prerequisite for PPD. For lesbian couples, there are often additional confounding factors, including the emotional and financial burden of in vitro fertilization, deciding who will do what, and jealousy or resentment when plans change.

Other issues contributing to depression in partners of all genders include increased financial stress and responsibility, sleep deprivation, lifestyle changes resulting in loneliness and isolation, and feeling emotionally, physically, and sexually neglected.

Partners often feel as though they have to be strong for the birthing parent. Usually, they feel as though they are the last one on the list to have their needs met. Think about it: So much of our energy goes into keeping this helpless newborn alive. We take it for granted that the non-birthing adult in the home can take care of themselves.

Although this workbook emphasizes birthing people suffering from PPD, please know that many of the tools here are useful for all parents. Above all, please also prioritize the mental health of partners. Partners, if you feel guilty taking up space or resources, think of getting help as putting on your oxygen mask. You need to take care of yourself first so you can take care of your family.

You *Can* Feel Better

The next part of this workbook dives into specific tools and strategies that can help you overcome PPD. When you are a new parent, you want help to feel better, and you want it fast.

The tools I've picked are based in CBT, which is widely shown to improve and prevent PPD. What is even better is that CBT has shown to be effective when used in alternative formats, like this workbook.

As you settle into the working stage, remember to be gentle with yourself. Many of these strategies may be foreign to you. We are trying to create new habits of thought. Starting a new habit is almost always hard at first, but the more you practice it, the easier it becomes.

I am hopeful that you, like so many of my clients, will start to internalize the positive reframing that CBT teaches. In time, a happier and more positive outlook will come naturally.

Part 2

Tools and Strategies

You are here because you want to feel better—and quickly. Understanding postpartum depression (PPD) and other perinatal mood and anxiety disorders (PMADs) is important, but insight alone may not provide all the help you need. In this part of the book, you will find practical tools and strategies you can start using right away to bring about lasting relief.

PPD impacts us in many different ways. To help you find the appropriate solution and strategy, I have organized this part into four color-coded sections:

Tools and Strategies for My Thoughts (pages 25–43). This section will help you identify your automatic thoughts, notice how they shape your beliefs, and learn how beliefs may be magnifying your symptoms of PPD. If we can notice something isn't totally true and challenge it, we might feel better.

Tools and Strategies for My Feelings (pages 44–54). In this section, we will look at tools you can use to improve your mood, cope with difficult feelings, and find relief *fast*.

Tools and Strategies for Relationships (pages 55–69). In this section, we will dive deeper into relationships with others, especially your romantic and/or coparenting partner. Your relationships change greatly after the birth of a baby, but they are even more crucial to your ability to get through this challenging time.

Tools and Strategies for Self-Care (pages 70–94). Self-care tools and strategies will not only help you get through the postpartum stage and manage the symptoms of PPD, but they will also help you thrive as you transition to parenting a toddler and, later, an older child. These tools and strategies will also help you retain a little bit of space inside you for you. Let's support your overall well-being, highlighting the activities and things that bring you joy and help you recharge.

Feel free to jump ahead to the topic or issue that most concerns you. I encourage you to find at least one tool to try out *today*.

Negative Filters

When we have PPD, our beliefs tend to be more negative. We often are overly critical of ourselves and pessimistic. If you are experiencing this thought pattern, please don't judge yourself.

Have you ever heard the phrase "looking through rose-colored glasses"? PPD slaps glasses tinted dark gray over our view. Everything gets filtered more negatively.

Fortunately, it is possible to start to correct a negative filter. The first step is noticing it.

Here are some common negative filters (called cognitive distortions because they distort our cognitions, or thoughts) that many postpartum women experience. Check off the ones that apply to you, even if just occasionally.

☐ The Shoulds

Many new parents have unrealistic expectations of what they *should* be doing, how their partners *should* be acting, or how their babies *should* be developing. Try to watch out for things you say to yourself starting with "I should . . ." For example, "I should know what to do by now," or "My baby should be sleeping through the night." Such statements are likely to make you feel more depressed and anxious. Quite likely, they aren't even true. (This is one reason joining a new parent group can be helpful. It can challenge some of the unrealistic expectations you consciously or unconsciously are struggling with.) Please don't *should* all over yourself.

☐ All-or-Nothing Mamas

This is a common mental filter for new moms. If you have previously been high-achieving in your career or education, you may have gotten used to doing it all. I'll let you in on a secret: There is no "doing it all" as a parent. Whether you stay at home, work from home, or work outside the home, there is simply no way to accomplish everything or be a perfect parent. If anything less than perfection is failure for you, you will really struggle with your mental health postpartum.

☐ Catastrophizing

Does your mind tend to go to the worst possible scenario? As parents, we prioritize keeping our babies safe. But how often do you think about extreme situations? Perhaps this comes from a reality-based fear after your child was in the NICU or because your child has special needs. However, if your thoughts are going to unrealistic extremes, you might be prone to catastrophizing.

☐ Mind Reading and Fortune Telling

Do you imagine what others are thinking (especially negative things about you)? Could you be overly anticipating judgment? Do you speak or act based on what you assume others will say? Are you predicting what will happen (especially bad things)?

☐ Mom Is Always Right*

Do you know the best way to diaper and soothe your baby? Can your partner never seem to do it as well as you? Do you jump in and take care of things because your partner doesn't do them correctly? Unfortunately, your partner won't get comfortable caring for the baby if they never have a chance to practice. How about being right during disagreements? Do you find you have to prove your point, even at a cost to your relationship? Do you defend your perspective even when it means your happiness suffers?

Not just a mom thing—all parents do it!

☐ Overgeneralizing

New moms with PPD are vulnerable to blowing up one bad event into a never-ending pattern. When the nights are long and the endless days seem monotonous, tedious, and hard, it is easy to fall into a trap of thinking the bad times will go on forever. Some parents might overgeneralize their performance. Watch out for statements that start with "I always . . ." or "I never . . ." or "You always . . . " or "You never . . . "

☐ Personalization

Personalizing is a cognitive distortion in which you assign an unreasonable amount of blame to yourself for things that are beyond your control. Sadly, I hear women say that it is their fault after they suffer a miscarriage or other perinatal loss. Even if they rationally believe that what happened was beyond their control, emotionally it feels as though they made a mistake or caused it to happen. (If you are in this boat, please accept my reassurance that it is not your fault!) Other parents may view perceived developmental differences in their baby as a result of their parenting; for example, "My baby can't roll over. It's my fault for not doing enough tummy time." (Again, not your fault.)

HOW ABOUT YOU?

Now go back and look through the negative filters you checked. Write the names of the filters here.

_____

_____

Which ones trip you up the most? Put a star next to those.

Next, can you think of an example of a distortion you experience or have experienced? Write it down here.

_____

_____

_____

Core Beliefs around Birth and Motherhood

Often, our negative filters are rooted in our core beliefs. These are things that we believe, even if they aren't true. They could be at the forefront of our mind or in our subconscious.

Read over the following common core beliefs others have around birth and becoming a mother. Identify ones you might have believed in the past, or still do. The belief may be something you rationally think isn't true but have still caught your inner voice saying.

Rate each belief by writing the corresponding letter on the line:

O = I think often   S = I think sometimes   N = I never think

"Getting pregnant is easy." _____

"If I'm healthy and doing everything right, I'll get pregnant." _____

"If I don't get pregnant, there must be something wrong with me." _____

"It's not fair that . . . (e.g., others get pregnant before me/have easier pregnancies/have more support/lose the weight faster)." _____

"Everyone else gets pregnant on the first try." _____

"If I miscarried, it must be from something I did wrong." _____

"Everyone else is glowing when pregnant, but I look bad." _____

"If I'm not all belly and thin everywhere else, I've gained too much weight and let myself go." _____

"If I have a C-section, I haven't had a natural birth. I've failed to give my baby the best start." _____

"Breastfeeding should come naturally." _____

"Women naturally know how to breastfeed and care for babies." _____

"If I can't soothe/feed/comfort my baby, what kind of mother am I?" _____

"Everyone else has everything all together." _____

"I hate my body." _____

"I should be enjoying motherhood; otherwise, I'm not a good mom." _____

"I'm damaged, defective." _____

"I'm unworthy, unlovable." _____

"No one understands." _____

Now write some of your own:

_____

_____

_____

Go back and take a look at the beliefs that you marked as ones you think *often*. What were they?

_____

_____

_____

_____

Please remember these negative core beliefs and be on the lookout for them. First, these thoughts aren't true—or at least, they aren't ALL true. Second, these thoughts are more likely to lead you down a spiral of depression and anxiety. Some people call them "monkey thoughts" or "stinking thinking."

Now that you are aware of them, you will be able to challenge them.

Challenging Automatic Negative Thoughts

Now that you have identified some negative core beliefs, let's talk about how they could impact you. Some new mothers find thoughts pop automatically into their heads, while others aren't as aware of their negative beliefs until they spend some time reflecting, journaling, or in therapy.

Here's an example of an automatic negative thought: "I'm failing as a mom."

Our goal is not only to recognize these as automatic negative thoughts, but also to start to challenge them. Each time you have a negative thought about yourself or your situation, can you challenge yourself to reframe it as a positive, or at least neutral, thought?

Some find it helpful to imagine a little devil on one shoulder whispering the negative thought. I like how this imagery distances the thought from one you are having and believing to one coming from outside of you—an unhelpful intrusion. Others call it their "monkey brain" or "monkey thoughts." The devil/monkey brain is often using negative filters. Go back to page 25 and make sure you aren't using one of the negative filters.

You could also picture an angel on your other shoulder, saying, "You are an amazing mom and here are five reasons why." Some parents like to picture their best friend or someone who cares about them offering positive comebacks to the negative thoughts.

If this is still too hard for you, try to simply shift, or reframe, an overly critical thought to a neutral or more balanced one. Then, back up the new thought with some evidence that supports the neutral or balanced thought.

Here is an example of how this works:

AUTOMATIC NEGATIVE THOUGHT	POSITIVE OR NEUTRAL REFRAME	EVIDENCE SUPPORTING THE REFRAME
"I'm failing as a mom."	"This is hard, and some moments I struggle, but I'm learning a little bit more every day."	→ I'm able to tell when he is hungry. → He's back up to his birth weight. → The pediatrician seemed to think he was okay. → He's grown out of his newborn clothes.

Now it's your turn to give it a try! Fill in the chart using the example as a guide.

AUTOMATIC NEGATIVE THOUGHT	POSITIVE OR NEUTRAL REFRAME	EVIDENCE SUPPORTING THE REFRAME

Using the ABCs of CBT

Let's review the ABCs of cognitive behavioral therapy (CBT), which we discussed in part 1 (see page 17).

When something happens or someone says something, it doesn't actually make us feel a certain way. It was simply the activating event. However, our beliefs about what happened, ourselves, and the world color, or influence, how we then feel.

Put simply, Activating events (A) *lead to* certain Beliefs (B) that *cause* emotional or behavioral Consequences (C). You can think of it as a progression, like this:

$$A \rightarrow B \rightarrow C$$

Want to see an example?

(Activating Event) Nia takes her baby to her six-month checkup. The pediatrician asks Nia why she hasn't started the baby on solids yet.

BELIEF	CONSEQUENCE
"I'm behind. I should've started solids already."	Nia might feel guilty and bad about herself as a mother.
"I'm failing as a mother. The doctor must think I'm not trying."	Nia might feel shame, embarrassment, or both.
"When did this doctor train? All the lactation specialists say not to rush solids until well after six months!"	Nia might be angry at the doctor or start to lose trust in his guidance.

Do you see how different beliefs lead to different consequences?

We cannot control activating events, but we *can* choose what we believe about them.

Thought Record

Thought records are a way of starting to notice how different beliefs make us feel. They are a very powerful way to then take control of our thoughts and feelings.

Let's use a new example.

*(**Activating Event**) Lupe is up in the middle of the night with a crying baby. She has checked his diaper and fed him and isn't sure why he's still crying.*

If Lupe's thoughts are colored by PPD, she might have one of these beliefs and its consequence.

BELIEF	CONSEQUENCE
"I don't know how to properly care for him. I'm failing as a mother."	Lupe feels bad about herself as a mother.
"I can't believe my partner isn't helping more. It's not fair."	Lupe feels anger and resentment.
"What's wrong with him? Why do I have to have the difficult baby?"	Lupe feels confused and might feel like a victim.
"He's never going to go to sleep. I am never going to get a good night's sleep."	Lupe feels hopelessness.

Lupe decides to challenge her beliefs. She comes up with a new alternate belief that is more hopeful, less critical of herself, and more neutral. Can you see how it leads to a more helpful emotional consequence?

ALTERNATE BELIEF	NEW CONSEQUENCE
"This is just what babies his age do. He will eventually grow out of it."	Lupe has acceptance and finds comfort knowing this stage will pass.

YOUR TURN

Can you think of a recent time you struggled?

What was the activating event?

_____

_____

Now think about what beliefs were underlying your feelings. Feelings, your emotional state or reaction, are sometimes confused with thoughts. Part of our work is uncovering the thoughts (or beliefs) that contribute to feelings, especially negative feelings, such as sadness, fear, and shame.

BELIEF	CONSEQUENCE

Next, I'd like to invite you to challenge yourself to come up with at least one or more alternate beliefs. Try to propose a positive, or at least neutral, explanation. It doesn't matter if you don't totally believe it yet. We are just experimenting with alternate beliefs. What could be the potential new consequence?

ALTERNATE BELIEF	NEW CONSEQUENCE

Want to try one more? Can you think of another recent example?

BELIEF	CONSEQUENCE

ALTERNATE BELIEF	NEW CONSEQUENCE

Sit for a moment with what you wrote under *alternate belief* and *new consequence*. What does that feel like? Did that shift make a difference? Write down your reactions.

Scary Thoughts

Good Moms Have Scary Thoughts is the name of a book by Karen Kleiman and Molly McIntyre, illustrated with true secrets submitted by real people. The premise is that many of us feel too ashamed or embarrassed to express anything other than enjoyment of motherhood. We fear judgment, keep our dark thoughts secret, only post happy photos to social media, and therefore reinforce the idea that everything is fine.

But many parents have thoughts that are more upsetting. It is not unusual postpartum to have intrusive thoughts of accidentally, or even intentionally, hurting your baby or someone else.

Remember, you are not your thoughts. True, women with PPD, anxiety, and OCD sometimes have thoughts about harming their child or others, but this is very different from having a serious plan or intent to hurt someone.

Why do we have scary thoughts? My theory is that the scary thought is our worst fear. Typically, the clients I work with love their children and families and would never want anything bad to happen to them. The intrusive thought is more like a worry or a fear. Anxious people have bright and creative minds. The scary thought is your brain's way of preparing for the worst-case scenario and helping you stay safe.

Unfortunately, fear of stigma keeps many postpartum women from speaking up. Some mothers fear their children could be removed from their care, while others simply fear being judged.

However, if we share our distressing and disturbing thoughts, it takes the power away from the secret. Check out the hashtag #SpeakTheSecret on social media. You will quickly see you are not alone.

BREAK THE SPELL

If you feel this workbook is a safe and private place for you, this activity is an invitation to deflate the power of your fears by writing them down. Remember, intrusive thoughts of doing something scary are *not* the same thing as planning or intending to do it.

What are you afraid of doing? What scary thoughts have come into your head?

What did it feel like to write down your scary thoughts?

What do you think it would it be like to share what you wrote with someone you trust?

_____

_____

If you were to share what you wrote with someone, who would it be?

_____

_____

What might be the benefit of sharing your scary thoughts?

_____

_____

_____

If your scary thoughts are intrusive and not an actual risk, please take this section as reassurance. However, I do recommend talking with a therapist or other provider about ways to manage these thoughts and gain support.

Stop Terrorizing Yourself

We've talked about negative thoughts and core beliefs. But what about thoughts that prey on your worries and fears?

Postpartum depression is often an anxious depression. Many women feel like they can't stop worrying about their baby.

I'll share a real-life example I experienced as a new mom. Whenever I drove anywhere, I worried about getting into a car accident. It was one thing to be in an accident as a young adult, but quite another now that someone depended on me. I started thinking about what would happen if I was hit by another car and ended up in a coma. Next, I started worrying about whether the hospital would know I was breastfeeding and if they would hook me up to a breast pump. Then I imagined losing my hard-earned milk supply. Next, I started worrying about the fact that I didn't have enough life insurance. Like a movie playing in my head, I pictured my husband learning about my death and my child growing up without a mother.

Usually, by that point, I recognized my thoughts were headed down a very unhelpful track. Unfortunately, by then, my nervous system had kicked into fight or flight mode, and it was hard to relax.

Do you ever find your worries spiraling? If so, try the following strategy.

STOP THE TRAIN AND CHANGE TRACKS

This exercise is useful for both perinatal anxiety and depression. When you notice yourself going down a worrying track:

1. Notice what you are doing. Are you terrorizing yourself with your thoughts? A little bit of worrying can be productive if it helps us to prepare. Are your thoughts productive or just bothering you?

2. If your thoughts are bothering you, decide to stop the worry train and change tracks.

3. Shift your focus onto something else. Distraction, such as music, TV, or calling a friend, is totally acceptable at times like this.

4. If you aren't sure if a thought is really a pressing fear, run it past someone you trust. If your confidant reassures you, accept their reassurance. Ultimately, I want you to be able to differentiate real, immediate threats from anxiety, but, initially, you can do a reality test with someone who has your back.

Your Reproductive Story

Your reproductive story refers to the vision or dream you have held in your head about having children, perhaps since childhood. Maybe it is something you said aloud: "I want to get married and then have two children, either a girl and a boy or two girls. I'm going to be a loving mom and meet all their needs." Or maybe it was something you didn't think about too concretely, but you just assumed motherhood could be an option. Maybe your desires and wishes have changed over the years.

Let's take some time to reflect. Write the earliest reproductive story you can remember. How old were you? What informed it? Where did you get the ideas of what you wanted and didn't want? Did your story feel realistic to you? Did you imagine it would come true?

When Your Reproductive Story Becomes a Nightmare

Regardless of how conscious you were of having a reproductive story, as described previously, you almost certainly had one. And I'm willing to bet you never planned on any of the following:

→ "I'm going to have five miscarriages."
→ "I'll have an abortion at 19, then when I can't get pregnant years later, I'll blame myself."
→ "I'm going to suffer from indecisiveness, never knowing when the right time is to start a family."
→ "I'm going to have postpartum depression and constantly think I'm a horrible mom."
→ "I will survive years of infertility treatments, only to feel unattached to the baby I ultimately have."
→ "I'll conceive after a stillbirth and be wracked with anxiety throughout the pregnancy."

Okay, you get the picture. I'll stop scaring the pregnant readers.

Alternatively, you could experience a small loss or shift from the vision you had for your reproductive story. Perhaps you planned an unmedicated birth and ended up having a C-section. Some people will tell you, "All that matters is that you have your baby." I'm going to tell you that it does matter. Any variance from your reproductive story is a loss. In fact, it is often loss on top of loss, on top of loss.

What we need is to hold space for our losses and take the time to grieve.

Reproductive Loss Is a Disenfranchised Grief

Disenfranchised loss refers to one that isn't always seen or recognized. It isn't publicly mourned. People don't know what to say in response to disenfranchised grief, such as for perinatal loss. They may not even know you suffered a loss or had difficulty conceiving, as many couples keep infertility a secret.

You might feel like others minimize your loss, set a time limit for how long they expect you to be impacted, or pressure you to get over it.

When someone loses a grandparent, they are sad, but they have rituals in place to mark the life and death of their loved one. Your work has an established bereavement leave policy for such a loss. People know what card to buy, what ceremony to plan, and how to be supportive and gather. On the other hand, many people feel awkward when they hear about infertility or miscarriage and will sometimes avoid you, leaving you feeling even more isolated. At such times, the birth announcements and baby showers of your friends can feel intrusive or even inconsiderate.

Similarly, if you are grieving the loss of your ideal birth plan, you may be surrounded by others telling you to be grateful you have a live baby. I'm here telling you it's okay to grieve the loss of your expectations. In fact, it is essential that you do.

DIVING DEEPER

This tool is a doozy, so take as much time as you need for it. Take breaks and practice self-soothing if you find it's too triggering.

Write your actual reproductive story. What has been your journey? Include your birth story, if you have any. Be as detailed as possible and include your feelings then and now. Take breaks writing this as needed, practice extra self-care, and have people around to support you.

When you're done, can you now read your story with gentleness? Imagine it is the story of a friend. Would you hold space for their grief? Would you gently challenge them if they blamed themself unfairly? Can you now do the same for yourself?

Your Story Continues

Quick check-in: Are you feeling okay? You are doing a great job processing some difficult stuff. Want to take a break? That's okay! Come back after you have done a little self-soothing. Because your story continues.

And we are glad that it does.

Once, I knew someone who had a string of bad luck. She felt like she couldn't catch a break and she told me she felt as though her life was a soap opera. I told her, nah, she wasn't a soap opera person. She was in a novel. She happened to be at the part of the story when it seemed darkest. I asked her, "What happens next?" Because there was certainly more story to come.

You are in the middle of your reproductive story. It doesn't end here.

Where will your story take you? Imagine where your story goes from here. How does your character overcome the challenges? How are they transformed by the journey? Where do they end up? How do they take the time to grieve loss and be aware of trauma *and* also be aware of joy and happiness? Can you envision the potential for growth as a result of all that has happened?

Always remember, it gets better. Your story continues!

Yes, And . . .

And now for something completely different!

My cousin is an improv comedian. She's good. In fact, she quit her day job several years ago and makes her living teaching and performing long-form hip-hop musical improv in New York.

In addition to demonstrating how saying "boots and cats" is the secret to beat-boxing, she blew my mind the first time she explained the number-one rule of improv: "Yes, and . . ."

If you are in an improv scene with a partner and they say you are both on the bus, you never say, "No, we are at the grocery store." In order for the scene to work, you always say, "Yes, and . . ." For example, "**Yes**, we are on the bus, **and** we are on our way to the zoo."

Being the therapy nerd I am, I immediately applied this technique to my counseling work with clients. This is how we overcome trauma. Healing happens when we can say, "*Yes*, something bad happened, *and* I am okay today" or "*Yes*, I grieve for what happened, *and* I have hope for the future."

Here are more examples:

YES	AND
I had a difficult birth.	I can grieve my birth plan and be grateful my baby and I survived.
I can be grateful for what I have.	I can still think this season of life stinks.
I have absolutely no idea what I'm doing as a parent.	I think the kids are going to be all right.
I'm totally overwhelmed.	I have moments of joy.
I'm glad I have time at home with my family.	I miss going out with my friends.

A dual awareness helps us to hold in our head two seemingly conflicting ideas. My goal with this tool is for you to start to develop this dual awareness.

I don't believe we move past trauma by forgetting it. I want you to get to a place where you can say, "Yes, and . . ."

Now it's your turn. Try to come up with a few of your own.

YES	AND

The Mood State Pyramid

In order to improve your mood, it is helpful to first better understand and observe it. This exercise will give you some tools for tracking your PPD.

First, let's establish some common language for your moods. Take a look back at the Mood State Pyramid on page 7.

Feeling depressed means different things to different people. You might hear people say, "I feel depressed." For some, it means they are feeling a four on the pyramid, while others may be trying to describe a one.

Using the pyramid, what range of numbers best represents how you felt this week? _____

Today? _____

The most extreme in your life? _____

What Is "Normal"?

For the purposes of better understanding your PPD, it is helpful to remember that most people experience a range of moods from three to seven. For many people, mood swings within this range are not problematic.

"But I don't like feeling a three!" you might say. Stick around. This section will give you the tools and strategies you need to feel better.

If you feel a two represents how you have been feeling most days, you might want to start another form of treatment, such as therapy, in addition to this workbook.

If you are at a one, I encourage you to talk to your doctor about possibly starting medication, if you haven't already.

If you feel you are at zero, please access support from a hospital emergency room immediately. In the United States, the National Suicide Prevention Lifeline is 1-800-273-8255, or call 911. The crisis text line is available 24/7 in the United States and Canada (text 741741). International hotlines are listed on SuicideStop.com.

What About the Ups?

Any kind of manic episode is more concerning postpartum than it is at other times in our life. Postpartum mania can lead to postpartum psychosis. Please check in with your doctor if you have days when you feel at an eight or higher.

Daily Mood Log

Now that we have a common language about feelings, let's start to track those feelings. Keeping a record of your highs and lows will help you get a better picture of your PPD. You might end up being surprised by your pattern.

For each day, write your mood as a number, from 0 to 10. Refer to the Mood State Pyramid as needed. If you feel your mood changed throughout the day, feel free to record the range, for example, "3–4" or "2–6."

	SUN	MON	TUES	WED	THUR	FRI	SAT
WEEK 1							
WEEK 2							
WEEK 3							
WEEK 4							

Once you have tracked your mood for a month or so, take a look. Are there any patterns?

_____

_____

_____

Are you comfortable with the pattern of your moods? Or would you like to make some changes? How?

_____

_____

_____

If you are seeing a provider for your perinatal mood or anxiety, I recommend bringing this log to your next appointment.

Opposite Action

When you're feeling down, it can be really hard to feel motivated to do the things you've been avoiding. Using the opposite action strategy can make it a little easier.

What is opposite action? The concept comes from dialectical behavioral therapy, which combines CBT with some of the mindfulness concepts of Zen Buddhism. It is a deliberate attempt to do the opposite of what your emotions urge you to do.

Here are some examples:

→   Forcing yourself to get up and go outside when all you want to do is stay in bed.
→   Facing your fear and that thing you have been avoiding.
→   Reaching out to new mom friends when you feel like withdrawing socially.
→   Taking a shower and doing a little extra grooming when you are feeling "blah."
→   Eating something small when you are nauseated (this one I mastered during an extended run of severe morning sickness).

What forms of opposite action would you like to try?

Postpartum Anger

Oh, anger—the PPD symptom we least expect. Many women experiencing postpartum anger might not even realize they have PPD. Some women will externalize their anger or attribute it to outside sources. Often partners will get the brunt of the misplaced anger. Other postpartum parents might feel angry at the baby for waking them up, being difficult to soothe, not feeding easily, or just disrupting their lifestyle.

Many with PPD may recognize that their angry, or even rageful, reactions are out of proportion or misdirected, but still feel unable to control their reactions. Unfortunately, this can also lead to a cycle where we blame or judge ourselves for the outburst. This can lead to embarrassment, shame, hopelessness, and feeling out of control, which leads to depression. The depression then predisposes us to more anger, putting us in a vicious cycle:

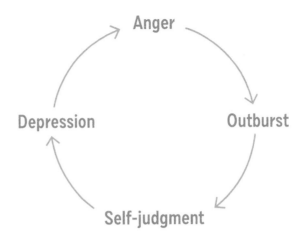

Parents of all genders can experience PPD as anger. In fact, depressed male-identified parents are more likely to express anger than feel sad, as they may have grown up thinking anger is more socially acceptable than being weak or vulnerable.

However, more female-identified parents have been raised and socialized to be nice. Internalized misogyny and cultural stereotypes around being "bitchy" may increase shame and embarrassment over angry outbursts, which may feel like PMS on steroids.

In fact, hormones do play a role. From an evolutionary standpoint, your body may be trying to prioritize your new baby by keeping a partner away from you so you won't get pregnant again too soon. This may seem more obvious for heterosexual, cisgender relationships, but LGBTQIA families also report that one or more parents feel their hormones have shifted away from sex and romance and toward growing and caring for the baby through cuddling or chest-feeding.

THE ANGER FUNNEL

You may have heard that anger is a secondary emotion. But what does this really mean? I like to use the visual of a funnel, with other primary emotions funneling down from the top and feeding the experience of anger.

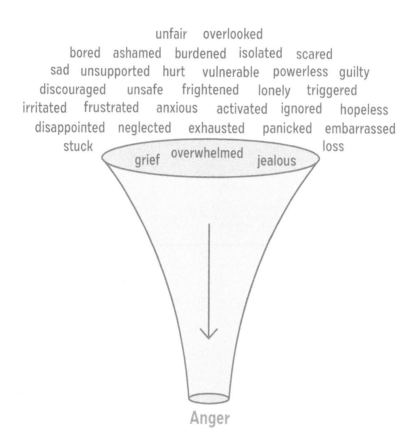

Circle the feelings that could be feeding into your anger funnel.

What feelings, if any, would you add to the top of the funnel?

_____

_____

Which feelings are most relevant or difficult for you?

_____

_____

How could you begin to address the underlying emotions contributing to your postpartum anger?

_____

_____

You might also be feeling seemingly positive feelings along with negative ones. This is normal, but it can be disorienting and confusing. Or, it may make you feel like the negative feelings aren't justified.

Might you simultaneously be having any of these feelings?

→ Excitement
→ Love
→ Enjoyment
→ Relief
→ Joy

It is okay not to know exactly how you are feeling. It is okay if all you can say currently is that you are having feelings. Being able to name your feelings can come later, upon reflection.

Remember, many women with PPD experience anger and rage. To reduce stress, try practicing the tool in the next exercise, as it works equally well with anger.

But most of all, please don't judge yourself. Instead, focus on how your body is inviting you to pay attention to your needs.

Emotional Flooding (aka the Fight or Flight Response)

You may have noticed at the end of the last exercise on anger that I mentioned your body is inviting you to pay attention to your needs. I think anger, trauma, and anxiety (and most strong emotions) are basically the same thing.

What is more, these feelings are not just in your head. They are in your body, especially your nervous system. Have you ever heard of the fight or flight response? It is the autonomic nervous system (a part of your central nervous system) switching over from the parasympathetic nervous system (rest and digest) into the sympathetic nervous system (fight or flight). When your brain registers any kind of threat or anything reminiscent of a threat, your nervous system thinks it's helping you survive by switching over.

Once upon a time, when threats to our ancestors were more likely to be bears or saber-toothed tigers, the ability to run away quickly or pick up a club and fight off the predator was adaptive. Our ancestors were the ones who survived these threats and passed on this adaptation to us.

Let's look at the stress response in more detail.

Imagine a cave woman sitting in her cave, calmly using her hands to carve a new tool. She has just eaten a meal, which is digesting in her belly. Suddenly, a bear shows up at the mouth of the cave.

The woman's brain registers the bear as a threat, like an alarm bell sounding. Next, the fight or flight response shoots the stress hormones, epinephrine (adrenaline) and cortisol, into her body. Several bodily systems change to help her survive. Her body has decided that the tool she is carving will not matter if she dies, so the blood rushes from her fingertips into the large muscles in her legs so she can run. Likewise, there's no point using the advanced problem-solving part of her mind or digesting her meal if she's about to become one, so both processes stop to send resources elsewhere. Her heart starts pounding quickly to push extra blood throughout her body, and her lungs switch from slow, deep abdominal breaths to fast, shallow chest breathing.

Well done for the cave woman! The super-mellow cave people were eaten. This cave woman, quick to react, survives to have descendants—us. The fight or flight response, coming from the oldest reptilian part of this woman's brain, was quite adaptive to her needs.

Unfortunately, evolution is slow. Our nervous system still works in the same way today, but the threats we encounter are dramatically different.

Occasionally, you may hear of a mother who lifted a car off her trapped child. Adrenaline gave her the extra strength she needed in that moment. But what if the threat to her baby is a congenital heart condition? Will punching out the neonatologist improve her situation? What if she picks up her child and runs out of the NICU? Clearly, the stress response is maladaptive to most modern stressors.

Yet our bodies fire off these same ancient stress hormones. Worse, the stress hormones make it harder for us to think calmly, connect with others, or respond strategically.

In addition, the stress response was intended for occasional situations and only for short bursts of time. Imagine our modern NICU mother. The alarm bell of the cardiopulmonary monitor may sound several times a day. No big deal. Just the baby's heart or breathing stopping. Each time, a team of nurses rush in to prevent the real threat of fetal demise. Alarms sound all throughout the day and night, for days or weeks on end. The new mother's nervous system responds to the alarm bell each time, as well as to the alarms of the other babies in the NICU. And when her baby is finally discharged home, she remains vigilant for the real threat of the baby dying.

Perhaps her baby will need additional surgeries. Or perhaps seemingly innocent events, such as a neighbor child leaning in to kiss her baby's face, will feel life-threatening.

Our bodies are simply not wired for this kind of sustained, chronic stress. Over time, it negatively impacts our physical and mental health, leading to heart disease, weight gain, and PTSD.

Gosh, that sympathetic nervous system was just trying to help. If only there was a way to shut off that automatic response.

Have you ever tried to stop panic or fear? What worked and what didn't?

Have you tried telling yourself, "There is no scary bear"? (Or, "My baby won't die," or contradict whatever triggered you?) Perhaps it worked. But for most of us, simple self-talk cannot reverse a strong fight or flight response.

This is because you are only telling your brain. We need to give our *bodies* the all-clear signal.

What if I told you there *is* a way shut off the fight or flight response?

Your breath.

Although breathing is an involuntary function, we can voluntarily and purposefully change the *way* we breathe. Your breath is literally the off switch for the stress response.

SHUT STRESS OFF

Place one hand on your chest. Place the other hand over your belly button. Take a slow, deep breath. Which hand moved more?

If the hand on your chest moved more, try another deep breath, but this time, feel your belly button pull away from your spine as your abdominals expand with the inhalation.

Continue slow, deep breaths, feeling your diaphragm expand.

Inhale slowly, exhale completely. (And repeat as needed.)

There. You are manually overriding the fight or flight response and sending your body back into the relaxed state.

You can even combine the breathing with a mental message, such as "Everything is okay." What message do you most need to hear?

_____

_____

Now place one hand on your belly button and one hand on your back. The hand on your back should be roughly the same level as the hand on your belly button. Take another deep abdominal breath. Can you feel your back expand subtly as you breathe in?

If that didn't work for you, imagine you are wearing a pair of pre-pregnancy high-waisted jeans. As you breathe in, feel your breath push the waistband of your jeans out in the back as well as the front.

Congratulations! You are now using your diaphragm to push on the vagus nerve, which is a key player in your central nervous system, especially in recovery from the stress response. The vagus nerve will back you up when it's time for the relaxed mode.

Modeling Emotional Regulation for Our Children

This tool can help you manage your emotions. By using it in front of your child, you can motivate them to use it, too. If your baby is older than 12 months or if you have older children, start doing it right away for their sake.

The trick: Treat yourself like a toddler.

If your child is starting to melt down, you might suggest they take a time-out or practice something to regulate, such as a bubble breath (see below). For young children, I recommend taking the time-out with them. You might give them a hug, change locations, get some distance from the problematic toy or person, and give them some time to get calm.

A "bubble breath" is a simple way to lead a child in a deep, calming breath. As you breathe in, raise both arms above your head using an arc movement (like you're creating a bubble); as you exhale, bring your arms back down.

How do we get children to do something? We do it ourselves! Model how taking a break and doing bubble breaths helps you. This is super helpful when you find yourself getting frustrated with their tantrums. Wouldn't you rather they mimic us taking deep breaths instead of imitating our less healthy moments?

So often, we feel we have to have it all together or pretend to be calm and happy all the time. I say, show your kids you are human. Don't give them the impression you don't have bad moments. Instead, give them the gift you might not have had: emotional intelligence at a very young age.

Tell your child, "Mommy is feeling frustrated/angry/mad/sad right now. I'm going to take a bubble breath." Take a couple of big bubble breaths (including the arm movement) in front of them. They can copy you if they want, but don't force it. The important thing is that you do the breaths. Then tell your child how you feel: "That helped a little."

If you feel very overwhelmed or angry, role model taking a time-out as something you *want* to do. In my home, it is important to me that time-outs are not a punishment, but rather something we can all choose to take when we need it.

Postpartum Body Image

Our children are listening when we talk badly about our bodies. Although kids of all genders are learning how to value and respect women's bodies, female-identified kids are especially vulnerable to negative body comments.

LOVING ON MY BODY

Can you come up with five affirmations, or positive statements, about your body?

If this is challenging, think about what your body has done and can do. As your children grow up, try not to emphasize how they look to others, like they're an object to behold in the gaze of another. Raise your children of all genders to appreciate what their strong and growing bodies can do.

Your children will learn to love their bodies by hearing how you talk about your body. Start positive modeling here with statements you wouldn't mind them hearing and internalizing.

1. _____

_____

2. _____

_____

3. _____

_____

4. _____

_____

5. _____

_____

Now comes the fun part. Affirmations work best when we say them out loud to ourselves and repeat them. Make a copy of your list and tape it to your bathroom or bedroom mirror. Look yourself in the eyes and say your list out loud five times each day.

> **TIP:** It doesn't matter if you don't believe in the affirmations right now. Saying the affirmations over and over slowly brainwashes you into believing what you *want* to believe.

Social Support Assessment

First, let's take a look at all the important people in your life. Imagine yourself at the center of two concentric circles.

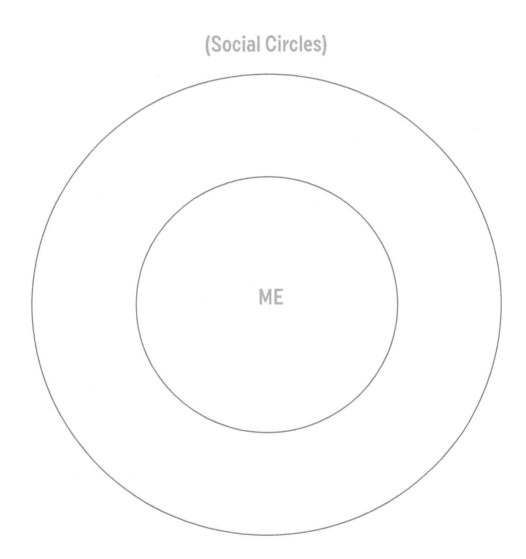

(Social Circles)

ME

Who is in the middle of your inner circle? A partner, other children, a best friend, parents, siblings? Write their names in the inner circle next to "ME".

The next layer, between the two concentric circles, represents the people who are just a little less close to you. Write down their names in this ring or layer.

Finally, around the perimeter, outside of both circles, write the names of people that are in your outermost layer. These should be people that are in your life but are not as close to you.

Now let's reflect.

What do you notice about the people in your different social support circles?

_____

_____

_____

How do you feel seeing your support in this way?

_____

_____

_____

What changes, if any, would you like to make? For example, do you need to bring in more support? Who could you rely on more? What relationships would you like to further develop or rekindle? Is there anyone toxic from whom you should distance yourself?

_____

_____

_____

Turning Toward Your Parenting Partner

If you have noticed a change in your relationship with your significant other postpartum, you are not alone. Two-thirds of couples experience less satisfaction in their relationship following the birth of a baby. In addition, PPD or anxiety in one or both partners can make the relationship worse.

If you and your child's other parent are no longer in a romantic relationship, I have news: You are still in a relationship. You are coparents. To be effective coparents for your child(ren), you will need even stronger communication skills. You have to do all the hard parts of a relationship without the rewarding bits. Although the tools and strategies for romantic intimacy may not apply to this relationship, take the time to read through the ones about communication and boundaries. You'll need them!

Note, this book includes ways to strengthen your relationship with your significant other. It is intended for people in relatively healthy relationships experiencing a dip in satisfaction following the birth of a baby. If you are currently in a relationship that is unsafe, please consider calling a domestic violence hotline. In the United States, the National Domestic Violence Hotline is available 24/7 at 1-800-799-SAFE (7233).

My single best tip for your relationship postpartum is to remember you and your partner are in this together. You are a team. You are not competing against each other.

Many of us feel a tremendous lack of time during this period. Babies need so much of our attention and energy around the clock. There doesn't seem to be enough time to attend to self-care, take care of the home, go shopping, work to make a living, and exercise. Many couples feel like it can be a competition or a contest to determine who is more deserving of time.

How well do you and your partner problem-solve the division of time and duties?

Grab your partner and your respective calendars for this next exercise. (Now is a great time to create a shared electronic calendar, such as an iCal or Google calendar, if you don't already have one.)

Think about a typical week. Designate a day of the week and time for *all* of the following:

Self-care for you: _____

Self-care for your partner: _____

Time to coordinate business, schedules, household chores, etc.: _____

_____

Time for relaxed family time together: _____

Time for enjoyable couple time: _____

When there is a scarcity of energy, support, and love flowing into the nuclear family system, it can sometimes feel as though you and your partner are competing for energy or draining each other. But it's not a competition when you can turn to each other.

There is a reason I listed self-care for each of you.

Imagine yourself and your partner as two cups filled with water. In a healthy relationship, when your water starts to go down, your partner can pour some water from their cup into your cup. Each of you can replenish the other's supply when it's running low.

However, if both of you are running low, it feels like more of a sacrifice to share any of your precious water—your energy, time, or love—with one another. Worse still, if you and/or your partner have a hole that drains your cup quickly—like PPD—trying to keep it full is a losing battle. The water will inevitably drain out of both cups.

But keep hope. Two whole cups overflowing with water can share water back and forth forever.

With this in mind, what are some ways you and your partner can replenish yourselves and each other?

_____

_____

_____

_____

_____

Warning Signs for Your Relationship After Baby

Relationship experts John and Julie Gottman have studied tens of thousands of couples over four decades. Their research sadly found that two-thirds of relationships suffer after the birth of a baby. Some of us can rebound, whereas other partnerships won't last. Having done so much research, the Gottmans found that they could predict which marriages would end in divorce based on just four characteristics.

Take this quiz to see if you and your partner could be at risk. I have written these questions to help you uncover if one of the Gottmans' warning signs is present in your relationship. Check off a statement if it applies to either one of you.

Risk Factor 1

Place a check mark next to the risk factor(s) you and/or your partner tend to do.

☐   We often start complaints with "You always . . . " or "You never . . . "

☐   It is important to discover who is right and who is to blame.

☐   Sometimes it's hard to stop the complaints once they start.

☐   We sometimes attack the other's character.

Scoring. If you checked off two or more statements, be mindful of *criticism* or verbally attacking personality or character.

The remedy to criticism? Try to use "I" language—that is, starting a statement with "I felt _____ [emotion] when _____ [objectively described incident] happened because I felt _____."
Rather than critique your partner's character, limit your complaints to one specific example. Better yet, rephrase your complaint as a positive request in the future.

Example. Instead of, "You never help me with the baby at night! You are so lazy and selfish." Try, "Could you get up with the baby the first time he cries after I go to sleep? I'm really struggling with sleep deprivation, and the first half of the night is the hardest for me to get up."

Still struggling? Try to "sandwich" one request for change between two compliments; for example, "Thank you for bringing me snacks when I'm breastfeeding. Next time, can you bring a larger glass of water instead of a juice glass? I feel so taken care of when you help me."

Risk Factor 2

Place a check mark next to the risk factor(s) you and/or your partner tend to do.

☐ Sometimes we lose respect for each other.

☐ One of us thinks, "I've felt disgust at times for my partner."

☐ Our fights involve sarcasm, eye-rolling, name-calling, or hostility.

☐ One of us feels morally superior to the other.

Scoring. If you checked off two or more statements, be mindful of *contempt*, or intending to attack or even abuse the other. Out of these four warning signs, contempt is the single biggest predictor of divorce.

The remedy for contempt? Build up respect, gratitude, and appreciation of each other. The Gottmans talk about "filling up the love bank" with lots of small gestures and kind words. They encourage a ratio of at least five positive interactions for every one negative interaction.

Example. "You're late getting home, again? Ugh. My sister said you'd never change. I'll never be able to count on you." Instead try, "Tell me about your day." (Really listen, too. Try to reflect on how they must have felt during the day.) Then ask if you can share. "I've been struggling this afternoon. The baby hit the witching hour and I just couldn't soothe her and make dinner at the same time. I know you are working hard to provide for us, but can you try to come straight home after work tomorrow? I really appreciate how you juggle everything."

Risk Factor 3

Place a check mark next to the risk factor(s) you and/or your partner tend to do.

☐ Say, "It's not my fault, you're the one who . . . "

☐ Shift the blame when hearing criticism.

☐ Often feel attacked, or like a victim.

☐ Feel like you are blamed too harshly for things going wrong.

Scoring. If you checked off two or more statements, be mindful of *defensiveness*. If you did, you and your partner are definitely not alone. Getting defensive is a very human response. The problem is that defensiveness defeats empathy and understanding. If you listen like a lawyer preparing a counterargument, you miss the chance to truly hear and understand your partner's point of view.

The remedy for defensiveness? Take personal responsibility. Try to walk in the other's shoes and see their perspective. Apologize if needed, then work together instead of against each other. Practice empathy and reflective listening.

Example. "What do you mean I bought the wrong diaper wipes? This is what you wrote on the shopping list! And why are you so particular anyway?" Instead try, "I'm sorry I got these wipes. Should we save them as backup? Next time, can we go over the shopping list together so we are clear?"

Risk Factor 4

Place a check mark next to the risk factor(s) you and/or your partner tend to do.

- ☐ Either one or both of you shuts down during arguments.

- ☐ Whenever conversations get hard, one of you stops out of fear of the conversation getting heated.

- ☐ One of you thinks, "It's better to say nothing at all than to say something to upset them."

- ☐ One of you says, "I can't say anything anyway, so just forget about it."

Scoring. If you checked off two or more statements, be mindful of *stonewalling*, which is when one partner completely withdraws emotionally, verbally, or physically to avoid conflict. Usually the person who withdraws is feeling emotionally flooded. (Remember the fight or flight stress response from the section on feelings?) Unfortunately, stonewalling often sets up a repeated pattern, with the stonewaller retreating or distancing and the other partner feeling frustrated, rejected, and pursuing the discussion. Relationship therapists call this the distancer/pursuer cycle, and it feels very frustrating to both partners.

The remedy for stonewalling and distancing/pursuing? Take a time-out so you can both calm down separately. This is an extremely useful tool for whatever trigger, emotion, or dynamic is flooding you. (We will take a closer look at time-outs next.)

Example. "Not this again. I don't want to talk about it." Instead try, "Honey, I'm feeling overwhelmed. Can we take a break for 20 minutes and try again? Or, if we're too tired, maybe this weekend during nap time? It's a hard subject, and I want to be feeling better when we attempt to talk about it."

Time-outs for Flooded Parents

You may have heard of time-outs in sports. They also work for relationships. When things are getting heated, either side can call for a time-out. Sometimes just 20 minutes of distraction is enough to help you come back together for a calm and more productive conversation.

Why do time-outs work? Because they give your flooded nervous system (see "Emotional Flooding" on page 49) some time to reset into a relaxed state. Here are some do's and don'ts for the time-out strategy:

→ Don't push to keep talking (or fighting) when your partner asks for a time-out. Respect the request.

→ Don't keep yourself worked up. For example, don't ruminate on the disagreement and keep yourself justified in your anger.

→ Don't take time to calm down without coming back to the disagreement. It will likely bubble up next time there is a slight tension.

→ Do ask for a time-out in a respectful way. Own it. Say *you* need some time to calm down versus blaming your partner for your feelings.

→ Do take some time to journal if you feel like you need to express yourself, get something off your chest, or remember what feels really important.

→ Do something to make yourself feel better.

→ Do come back to your partner. Maybe decide together ahead of time how long the time-out will be.

→ Do check in with each other by asking, "Are you ready to talk?"

→ Do set a time to have a productive conversation. Bring your journal.

→ Do revise and edit your journal. You don't need to read your partner every thought you had when you were angry. Think about what you really want and ask for it.

→ Do reconnect in a way that is meaningful for both of you, such as with a good hug.

Healthy Boundaries for New Parents

It never hurts to review healthy boundaries in general. As a therapist, I can give you a very unscientific statistic, my guesstimate, that at least 75 percent of people in therapy have room to grow in understanding how to maintain healthy boundaries. Becoming a parent will challenge your boundaries and your relationships more than ever, so let's review.

TYPES OF BOUNDARIES

Interpersonal boundaries are how you define and protect your personal limits. You can visualize them as a bubble or forcefield around you. Other people will make demands on your time, energy, and body as a new mom. It is crucial that you feel empowered to defend your needs.

Here are some other kinds of boundaries:

Physical Boundaries. Many mothers feel "touched out" by the end of the day. I like to empower breastfeeding mothers to set limits when they need to. Teach your children that your breasts are actually yours and not theirs, and that they need your consent to feed. This may sound strange, but infants as young as three to six months can understand and start to use baby sign language for milk. Start a habit of asking your children, and having them ask you, before you give your consent to start nursing. Respect your need to stop as well.

Sexual Boundaries. If you are among the one in three women who have a history of sexual abuse or sexual assault, be mindful of how triggering birth and mothering can feel. Honor your need to take breaks. Feel like you are in control of your limits. Find health-care providers that ask for consent before touching you. Postpartum intimacy may be more challenging, so make sure you are having open conversations with your partner.

Mental Boundaries. As a new parent, you will likely be inundated by opinions and judgment from others. Decide whose opinions about which topics really matter, then let the rest go. Act from your own values.

Social Boundaries. If you are an introvert, you will find it very hard to have such little time to yourself to recharge. If you are an extrovert and a social butterfly, you may find it challenging to be at home more and around your friends less.

In what ways have your boundaries been challenged since becoming a mother?

HEALTHY BOUNDARIES

The healthiest kind of boundary is one you define and control. Imagine yourself surrounded by a bubble with one door. The door can be opened and closed, but there is only one doorknob. Would you like the doorknob to be on the inside, controlled by you? (You could decide who to let in and when.) Or would you like it to be on the outside, controlled by someone else?

Boundaries

Healthy

Controlled by me

Unhealthy

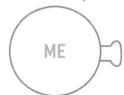

Controlled by another

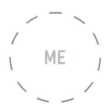

No doors or windows

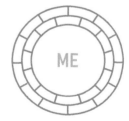

Walled in

Imagine the door to your house could only be opened by someone else. You could never predict or stop when someone opens it and comes in. Worse, what if there were no doors or windows?

People who have been abused in the past are more likely to have weak or damaged boundaries. But some go to the other extreme and build a brick wall around themselves so no one can get in to hurt them. Unfortunately, this means no one can get in to be with or help them, either.

If you have struggled with boundaries in the past, I'd like you to think about how you can prioritize your boundaries for the sake of your children. As with many things, children learn by example. Teach them from an early age about their bubble, your bubble, and where each bubble starts and stops. Let them know they are in charge of their own bubble and their own body.

Which kind of boundaries do you think you have?

How to Communicate Your Needs

Now that you have a better understanding of your boundaries and needs, ask yourself: How well do I communicate them? Let's look at aggressive versus assertive versus passive communication.

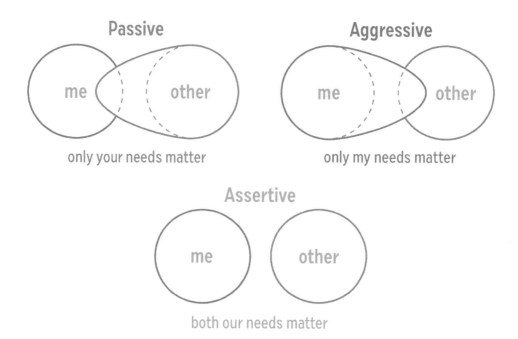

Many of the people I work with think being nice means respecting other people's boundaries—even at a cost to their own boundaries. I would love to help you see that you benefit others more in the long run if you also respect and defend your own boundaries.

Put another way:

→ Aggressive communication: Only my needs matter.
→ Passive communication: Only your needs matter.
→ Assertive communication: Both our needs matter.

Now let's rate your communication style. On the arrow below, mark an X to indicate how you are currently communicating your needs as a new mother:

←---→

Aggressive   Assertive   **Passive**

What do you think about your current communication style?

_____

_____

_____

Are there any changes you would like to make?

_____

_____

_____

Why would those changes be important?

_____

_____

_____

What would be the first steps you would take to change how you communicate?

_____

_____

_____

Postpartum Intimacy

Myth: A doctor will clear you at your six-week-postpartum visit as ready for sex.

Motherly's State of Motherhood survey results indicate that 31 percent of millennial women (defined as born from 1981 to 1996) reported resuming sexual activity after giving birth before feeling ready. In addition, 26 percent of women reported that sex was a significant stressor.

Does this surprise you? We live in the age of consent and #MeToo, but nearly a third of new moms are not communicating how they really feel about sex to their partners. Many OB-GYNs and midwives give a physical "all clear" to resume regular pelvic activities to new mothers at six weeks postpartum. But this permission in no way reflects how ready those new mothers actually are to resume those activities.

The Motherly survey also found that:

→ Fifty-three percent of women report becoming interested in sex again by six weeks after giving birth.
→ Eleven percent of women report becoming interested in sex again before six weeks.
→ Thirty-eight percent of women report it took 6 to 12 months before they were really interested in sexual intimacy again.

So if you are technically cleared, but not feeling it, you are in good company.

As a birthing parent, you may feel not ready physically for months as you continue to heal from tears, an episiotomy, a C-section, or other complications. Some mothers do not feel ready emotionally for even longer for reasons like not feeling comfortable or confident with their changed body, birth trauma, past sexual trauma that has been re-triggered, and sleep deprivation.

In addition, hormones play a large role in libido. Many birthing parents report being surprised at how long postpartum it takes to become interested in sex again. And don't forget about breastfeeding hormones, as the natural age of weaning can be anywhere from 2.5 to 4 or even 7 years.

Here's my theory: Your biological drive is directing you to focus your energy on your infant. Furthermore, your body wants you to avoid getting pregnant so you can nourish your nursling. This explanation makes sense for heterosexual couples. Lesbian and transgender couples also report the non-birthing partner feeling neglected sexually.

Sometimes new parents have all their nonsexual physical intimacy needs met by cuddling children. You may even feel "touched out" and have less desire to be near your partner. And some breastfeeders feel uncomfortable with sexual touch to their breasts.

Finally, hormonal birth control can have different and unexpected impacts on your libido postpartum than it did before your baby. Be sure to talk to your health-care provider about birth control options. You will ovulate before your first menstruation, which is why some families are surprised by a second pregnancy sooner than intended.

Male parents (both straight and gay) may be surprised to learn that their hormones change, too. Men may experience a drop in testosterone when their partner is pregnant or when they are bonding with a new infant. Lower testosterone levels frequently reduce libido. From an evolutionary perspective, the drive is no longer to sow their oats but to focus their attention on caring for their vulnerable offspring.

THE SIX-SECOND KISS

Are you ready to ease into feeling more intimacy and closeness with your partner? Regardless of whether you are ready to have postpartum sex, I do encourage more kissing. When was the last time you kissed for at least six seconds?

Many couples fall into a pattern where they have a quick peck at hello or goodbye. But kissing for longer is equated with foreplay. Unfortunately, if one or both of you are not in the mood for the whole shebang because it is too much of a production, you don't have the energy, or you just aren't ready, you might also be avoiding kissing. You might even tell your partner not to kiss you or flirt with you if you aren't ready to go all the way.

Sadly, we miss out on the benefits of kissing just for the sake of kissing. The early days of your dating probably involved making out and enjoying the pleasure of first base and the joy of flirting. By removing the association of kissing as foreplay, you can take away the pressure of whether kissing will lead to more and just have fun.

Try to kiss your partner every day for at least six seconds. That's how long it takes for oxytocin (the love hormone) to be released. Here's the challenge: Have a six-second kiss with your partner at least once a day for the next 14 days. Using the mini-calendar below, place a check mark on each day you do it. If you hate it, you can stop. But you might want to keep it up!

	SUN	MON	TUES	WED	THUR	FRI	SAT
WEEK 1							
WEEK 2							

Really not into kissing? Try a 60-second bear hug every day instead. Or you can measure a hug using three long breaths.

Grandma Advice

Let's get back to basics. I call this "grandma advice" for feeling better because it's not rocket science. It's the commonsense things you have surely heard before, the kinds of things a grandmother might suggest:

→ Get a good night's sleep (or take a nap)
→ Eat a bowl of chicken soup (seriously, almost every culture has a form of chicken soup, from "Jewish penicillin" to *caldo de pollo*)
→ Drink more water (especially if breastfeeding)
→ Avoid excessive alcohol and drugs
→ Surround yourself with people who love you
→ Go outside and be in nature or garden
→ Hug your baby, or pet your dog or cat

Can you be your own grandma? What commonsense improvements could you make to your lifestyle?

_____

_____

_____

_____

On a scale of 1 to 10, with 10 being the most important, how important do you think it is to make these improvements right now? Circle the number.

1   2   3   4   5   6   7   8   9   10

Why did you pick that number and not a lower one? Can you list five reasons it is important to make these improvements or how they may benefit you?

1. _____

2. _____

3. _____

4. _____

5. _____

Are there any barriers to making these improvements? If so, what are they?

_____

_____

_____

_____

How could you overcome those barriers?

_____

_____

_____

_____

Mothering the Mother and Matrescence

What underlies the concept of grandma advice? At its heart is the idea of being nurtured.

Part of the beauty—and the brutality—of the fourth trimester is your need to be cared for. But instead of being cherished and fed, you are doing the cherishing and feeding, 24/7.

Allowing yourself to be held, loved, and helped frees you up to honor the amazing period of personal growth you are experiencing. Our culture has baby showers, gender reveal parties, and dramatic pregnancy announcements. But how do we truly mark the birth of a mother?

As sacred and magical as your transition to motherhood is, it is also awkward, painful, and messy. *Matrescence* is a term that describes the developmental stage of becoming a mother. Similar to *adolescence* or the transition from child to adult, matrescence marks the transition from maiden to mother. We are hormonal and vulnerable, and we often go through an awkward stage before we can settle into our beauty and our new identities with grace and confidence.

Many mothers in individualist Western cultures are isolated. Living with just a partner and child(ren) separates new mothers from the aunties, mothers, big sisters, cousins, and friends who nurture new mothers in traditional village life, throughout the fourth trimester and beyond.

Are you nurtured and mothered? How, or how are you not? By whom?

What do you most need right now? How could you get that need met?

What do you most need to hear to feel loved and cherished? Write the words you most need to hear from a mother figure.

To Medicate or Not to Medicate

I encourage therapy and this workbook for mild to moderate PPD and anxiety. But there are times when antidepressant medication should be considered, such as for severe depression or symptoms that don't get better with therapy.

There are so many opinions about the use of antidepressant medication during pregnancy and breastfeeding. Perhaps you have a few of your own.

Reminder: This book is informational for PPD in general. It does not constitute medical advice and cannot replace the individual recommendations from your treatment providers.

My goal is always to support an individual's self-determination in regard to the decision to use medication. However, I am in a position to provide some research-based findings that can help you make an informed decision about what is best for you.

A reproductive psychiatrist is a medical doctor, board certified in psychiatry, who has advanced training and experience in treating perinatal mental health disorders. Some patients are also treated by psychiatric nurse practitioners and other prescribers who have a women's mental health specialization. (See the Resources section at the back of this workbook to find a treatment provider in your area.) Others start with their OB-GYN or midwife, especially if that person is someone they trust and can access easily. However, many OB-GYNs have never been trained in psychiatry, and many psychiatrists have never been trained in pregnancy or lactation. This double gap in knowledge highlights the need for expert advice from reproductive psychiatrists.

For those individuals who are currently taking an antidepressant for severe, recurrent depression and are trying to conceive, are pregnant, or are postpartum, most reproductive psychiatrists recommend that they stay on whatever medication works well for them. As many as 68 percent of women who stop taking an antidepressant in the perinatal stage relapse into more serious depression. If you are considering stopping the use of a psychiatric medication, please make an appointment with your doctor to talk it over before you take such action. Your doctor will have a personalized conversation with you about what has happened in the past when you have tried to stop taking an antidepressant.

If your antidepressant has been prescribed by a primary care doctor or psychiatrist less experienced with pregnancy and they are unsure of the potential risks during your pregnancy or breastfeeding, or if your OB-GYN feels your mental health is outside of their scope, you can get a second opinion from a reproductive psychiatrist or have your doctor call the PSI Perinatal Psychiatric Consult Line at 1-800-944-4773, extension 4. Additionally, either you or your provider can consult MotherToBaby for expert advice on the exposure of your specific medication to your baby during pregnancy and breast-feeding. Go to MotherToBaby.org or call 866-626-6847 or text 855-999-3525.

Some women fear that antidepressant use in pregnancy can lead to miscarriage, congenital abnormalities, cardiac malformations, autism, or long-term neurobehavioral effects. However, these fears have been shown *not* to be true risks. There are, however, very low increased risks (for less than 3 percent of pregnant women who take antidepressants) of preterm birth, low birth weight, and persistent pulmonary hypertension (PPHN). Yet, even these risks are hard to determine. Because guess what else causes preterm birth, low birth weight, and PPHN?

Untreated maternal depression.

That's right. As discussed in part 1 in "What Are the Risks of *Not* Treating PPD?" (see page 18), a pregnant woman's untreated depression is dangerous to her unborn baby's health.

It is a big decision whether to continue taking medication. Many of my clients are inclined to suffer, thinking being miserable is worth it, if it is best for their baby. (We can look at why I want you to ditch martyrdom later.) If your depression is severe and you would like to stay on or start an antidepressant, please consult a knowledgeable treatment provider.

For women who have a history of severe and/or recurrent depression or other mental health concerns, it can be helpful to be mindful of what could happen if medication is stopped.

If you are currently taking medication:

Have you gone off medication before? If so, what happened?

_____

_____

_____

_____

MEDICATION MYTH BUSTERS

There are a lot of myths about medication. Trust me, I've heard them all. There are many valid reasons to try other approaches before turning to psychiatric medication. But there is also a lot of bunk out there.

In this exercise, you're going to test your knowledge of fact versus myth. Read each statement while you use one hand to cover up the answer below. Circle *true* or *myth*, then read the answer.

1. Statement: "Antidepressants are addictive."

True   **Myth**

ANSWER: Addictive medications are those that create dependence and tolerance, or have a high risk for abuse. For example, certain medications for anxiety, like Xanax, Valium, Ativan, Klonopin, and others in the benzodiazepine family, can lead to tolerance. This means that if you take such medication regularly or take more than prescribed, you might need to take more and more to achieve the same effect. These fast-acting anxiety medications might be a good choice for occasional, severe anxiety, such as a panic attack, but they are not designed to be used on a regular, daily, long-term basis. In addition, there is some risk of anxiety rebound, where you feel even worse anxiety once the medication wears off.

Some antidepressants, on the other hand, are useful for anxiety in addition to depression. They are meant to be taken daily to lower the intensity of your symptoms so you can manage your PPD and anxiety using tools and strategies like the ones in this workbook.

A few antidepressants are known for causing headaches if you miss a dose or suddenly stop taking them. This is another reason to work with your doctor on a taper schedule when you want to stop, as opposed to quitting cold turkey on your own. However, the withdrawal is nowhere near the kind of withdrawal people experience when addicted to pain-killers, like opiates, or other drugs.

We are more concerned about the risk of addiction to painkillers and benzodiazepine anxiety medications because some people take them more than prescribed or for other reasons, such as to feel high or avoid life. Antidepressants do not cause a high that leads to abuse. So the answer is *myth*.

2. Statement: "If I see a psychiatrist, I will have to take medication."

True   Myth

ANSWER: Many reproductive psychiatrists are more than happy to support your choice to get off or stay off medication. They will want to develop a plan for how you will manage your PPD symptoms with-out meds, including a plan for sleep, social support, and therapy. Many like to check in with you regularly, for example monthly, to make sure you are on track. In addition, many of my clients like to do a consulta-tion session for the first visit, just to learn more about their medication options. There is never a commitment to start or stay on medicine. You are always in charge of this decision. So the answer is *myth*.

3. Statement: "There are some medications for mood disorders a pregnant woman should never take."

True   **Myth**

ANSWER: This one is true. Depakote, or valproic acid, for example, is a medication commonly used to treat the mood swings of bipolar II disorder. It is known to cause congenital malformations and lower the IQ levels of babies exposed to the medication in utero. Please take these scary side effects as reassurance that you will not be prescribed something so harmful.

4. Statement: "If you are taking medication during pregnancy, you should stop at the end so the baby won't get any of the medicine through breast milk."

True   **Myth**

ANSWER: This one's a myth. When you are pregnant, the baby is exposed to a much higher percentage of the medication through your bloodstream. However, a much smaller amount of medication is transferred through your milk. Frankly, stopping just before or just after birth is a rotten time to destabilize you.

5. Statement: "If you go on an antidepressant, you will have to stop breastfeeding."

True   **Myth**

ANSWER: Another myth. Just about every medication has a label saying, "Consult your doctor before taking if pregnant or breastfeeding." It can seem scary, but it's likely because there is such a scarcity of randomized control trials done with perinatal women. Please do go over your concerns with your doctor or lactation consultant, then accept their reassurance.

A variation of this one is, "If you take an antidepressant, you will have to pump and dump." Just, no.

6. Statement: "If I take meds, it means I'll end up like my aunt. I saw how they made her a zombie and overweight."

True   **Myth**

ANSWER: It is possible your family member had a different mental illness. The medications for psychotic disorders, like schizophrenia, or bipolar disorder that is difficult to manage are more heavy duty than antidepressants and cause more side effects, including weight gain. The goal of an antidepressant is not to numb you out or change your personality. You should feel like you are able to be yourself again, not like the meds are changing you. So the answer is *myth*.

7. Statement: "Antidepressants are just a Band-Aid. They don't solve any problems."

True   **Myth**

ANSWER: So, I'm going to go with *could* be true. This might be false for you if you are one of those people who has a chemical imbalance and no amount of exercise, self-care, or therapy has been able to alleviate your depression. However, if you are experiencing mild to moderate depression for the first time, only taking medication has the risk of being a Band-Aid if you then ignore the life issues underlying your depression, like a bad marriage or systemic injustice. Research backs up my clinical opinion that medication is not the best first choice for mild to moderate PPD. I would much rather someone start with therapy or a workbook like this one. For severe, dangerous, or debilitating symptoms of postpartum mental illness, I encourage a *combination* of meds and therapy.

How did you do?

0–3 RIGHT ANSWERS I'm glad you are here. These are common myths that a lot of people believe.

4–5 RIGHT ANSWERS You have been getting some mixed information, but you are on the right track.

6–7 RIGHT ANSWERS You are well informed. Start educating the people around you.

PROS AND CONS OF MEDICATION

If you have been on the fence about starting an antidepressant for PPD, use this next exercise to explore some of the potential risks and benefits. In the four quadrants on the next page, please list the following:

Pros of starting medication: List the potential benefits of starting an antidepressant.

Cons of starting medication: List all the bad things you think might happen if you start taking an antidepressant.

Pros of *not* starting medication: List the good things you think would come of not starting an antidepressant.

Cons of *not* starting medication: List all of the bad things that could happen if you do not start taking an antidepressant.

Decisional balance

	Starting medication	Not starting medication
PROS		
CONS		

Now go back through your pros and cons. Did you write down any myths? If something you listed is a myth—for instance, "I could get addicted"—cross it out.

Next, do you remember the negative filters we talked about in the "Tools and Strategies for My Thoughts" section (pages 25 to 43)? Go back through your lists and check if anything might be filtered by your depression; for instance, "I should be strong enough not to need meds," "It will mean I've given up," or "I should do it all on my own." If any of your statements might be overly filtered, please either cross them out or change them to something more neutral.

Take a look at the decisional balance. What do you think now?

_____

_____

_____

_____

Next step? If you think this is something to explore further, why don't you bring this exercise to your health-care provider? Please always tell your providers all your fears and concerns. Your fears and concerns are valid, even if I call them "myths." Talk about them. Always ask your questions. Please insist that your provider hear you and give you thoughtful responses. It is important to find a provider with whom you feel comfortable and who takes your questions seriously.

My Postpartum Coping Skills

Coping skills refer to the things you do to help you feel better and cope with stress and depression.

What's already working for you? You've gotten to this point, so you have to be doing *something that sustains you.*

Please make a list of the coping skills you are already using to good advantage.

_____

_____

Next, are there coping skills you have used in the past, or occasionally, that you would like to use more often?

Finally, are there any new coping skills that you would like to start or try? Brainstorm a list.

Look over these three lists. What action steps will be most important for you to take moving forward? In other words, think about the baby steps that will enable you to reach your new goals. What specific, measurable, and objective actions can you take?

Your Oxygen Mask

Have you ever flown on a plane? Do you remember the safety instructions before takeoff? On every commercial flight, there is an announcement that goes something like this:

> *In the event of the cabin suddenly losing pressure, oxygen masks will drop from the ceiling. If you are traveling with someone needing your assistance, be sure to secure your own oxygen mask first.*

Why do they always make a point of saying this? Because this statement goes against the instincts of most parents. Many parents would give the last of their own food or water to their child and go without.

The problem is, if you place an oxygen mask on your child first, then pass out yourself, you will not be able to help them.

How does all this tie in to your PPD? Essentially, I am asking you to be a little selfish and take care of your own needs first. It's the only way you will be able to help those who depend on you.

What "oxygen" do you need right now?

_____

_____

_____

On a scale of 1 to 10, with 10 being the most important, how important is it that you take steps to get this "oxygen"? Circle your answer.

1   2   3   4   5   6   7   8   9   10

Why did you select this number and not a lower one?

_____

_____

_____

If self-care sounds selfish to you, please think of it as something you are doing for others as well as yourself.

Remember, you can't pour from an empty cup. So keep your own cup filled!

GRAPES for Self-Care

Did you know a few GRAPES a day keep the psychiatrist away?

Everyone knows an apple a day keeps the doctor away. The vitamins and fiber in an apple are great for our physical health. But what about our mental health? Is there something simple to keep the psychiatrist away?

Why not try some GRAPES? I am not referring to the fruit, although grapes and grape products are delicious. I am talking about the acronym GRAPES:

Gentleness

Relaxation

Accomplishment

Pleasure

Exercise

Social

These elements help keep us happy and content and are ways to practice healthy coping skills. Use the acronym as a way to quickly remember activities you can do to practice self-care.

Let's get to know GRAPES:

GENTLENESS. Try to allow yourself to be gentle with yourself and your expectations. This might mean stopping the internal critic, forgiving yourself, or easing up on unrealistic expectations. This is a big one for many of the new parents

I work with. Especially if you have been successful in work or other areas of your life, it can be hard to suddenly be a novice in parenting.

RELAXATION. Make time in your schedule to do at least one thing you find relaxing. In your head right now, make a short list of your favorite relaxing activities. Do you feel guilty for taking a little time for yourself?

ACCOMPLISHMENT. Try to feel a sense of accomplishment at least once a day, either by crossing one thing off your to-do list or doing something really well. I believe everyone has at least one thing that they do very well or with mastery. What can you do? Don't be modest! You might take pride in the way you can change a diaper with just one hand. Or, you might find it meaningful to do things that were important to you before your baby.

PLEASURE. What activities truly bring you pleasure? You are entitled and deserve to have a pleasant mini-break each day. Do you treat yourself to at least one a day?

EXERCISE. Exercise is amazing, but please be realistic. If you just delivered a baby, think walking with the stroller or baby carrier, or simply stretching. Don't expect to go back to your pre-baby body instantly. However, did you know that 60 minutes of cardio exercise at least three times a week can be as effective as an antidepressant medication in lowering depression and anxiety? (If 60 minutes is more than you can do right now, aim for 30 minutes. Short periods of exercise can be helpful, too.)

SOCIAL. Make plans to ensure that you interact with positive people. Be mindful of your need to talk to others in this season of life or if you need to talk to someone about something other than babies.

BRAINSTORM YOUR GRAPES

Now let's brainstorm self-care activities for you! Some might be things you're already doing, whereas others might be activities you used to do but haven't done in a while. You might also like to add a few new things that you have never practiced but want to try.

Write down some ideas for each GRAPES element.

Gentleness:

_____

_____

_____

_____

Relaxation:

_____

_____

_____

_____

Accomplishment:

_____

_____

_____

_____

Pleasure:

Exercise:

Social:

GRAPES WEEKLY CHECKLIST

Have you had your GRAPES today? If you are feeling overwhelmed, depressed, anxious, or confused (or fill in your emotion), this checklist is a good place to start. Use it to document what GRAPES you do each day of the week. Make a check mark or draw a happy face or cluster of grapes (if you are more artistic than I) for each element you do, each day of the week.

	SUN	MON	TUES	WED	THUR	FRI	SAT
G							
R							
A							
P							
E							
S							

IMPORTANT: Keep in mind that a single activity can apply to more than one category. For example, walking in the park with a friend can be an Exercise, Pleasure, and Social activity. Daily perfection is not the goal. The last thing I want to do is add to your pressures and to-do lists. Rather, if you are feeling a little down, overwhelmed, or stressed, check in with yourself and see if any of the GRAPES could help you feel better.

GRAPES Accountability Partners

Have you ever started a new habit? How well did you stick with it? Creating new habits is hard for all of us.

Want to know what helps? Checking in with others. Maybe it's a little bit of (positive) peer pressure or maybe it's avoiding the embarrassment of having to tell someone we slacked off, but whatever the reason, accountability works. (There's a reason AA meetings and sponsors are helpful for so many in recovery.)

This next idea comes from a couple of friends who started texting each other every day after they started a daily exercise practice. Once they did their sit-ups and push-ups, they would text the other person: "Check, check." They swore it kept them more on track and for much longer than if they had been left to their own devices.

Rest assured, I am much more interested in developing your mental and emotional health than a six-pack or toned triceps. However, this simple idea inspired me to encourage my clients to find friends to be their GRAPES accountability partners. Now my clients message their group of mom friends and ask, "Have you done your GRAPES today?"

You and a friend could send a simple text with the letters done so far that day. For example, if you relaxed and were social, you could text, "RS." That's not so hard, now, is it?

Once you have introduced GRAPES to a friend or partner, you might be able to provide some needed perspective for each other. Perhaps if your friend or partner hears you being hard on yourself, they can remind you to practice Gentleness.

WHO CAN YOU SHARE GRAPES WITH?

Quickly jot down the names of a few people who might be good GRAPES accountability partners:

1. _____

2. _____

3. _____

4. _____

5. _____

Put a star next to the two or three who would be most likely to join you. Go ahead, text them right now and ask. No time like the present.

It will be harder to back out once you've put it out there. (That's the whole point.)

Mindful Meditation

Simply put, being mindful is the practice of turning your focus to the present moment. When we are worrying too much about the future, we can feel anxious. When we are dwelling on the past, we can feel depressed.

Mindfulness and meditation seem to be all the rage these days. But they've actually been around for thousands of years. There are many ways to practice them. Have you found something that works for you? Share it below:

If you have never done any mindful meditation, there are apps available to help you learn. (See a list in the Resources section at the back of this workbook.) Try starting with an app that helps you focus on your breath or do a simple body scan, like the one on page 109 ("Body Tension").

Have you had a mindful meditation practice in the past but find it hard to stay consistent? Great! That's the whole point! Stay with me. Mindfulness is not a state, a perfect Zen in which we sail through life unperturbed. It's the repeated turning of the mind back to our focus point.

It's the *process*, simply the trying and the desire. Every time you shift back from your automatic reactions, your sleepwalking, and mindless scrolling, you are flexing your mindful muscles in ways that will help your PPD and relationships.

As a therapist, I find that mindful meditation is often an important piece in helping clients heal from postpartum trauma, manage PPD and anxiety, and improve relationships.

My personal path of practicing started in college. I gravitated toward a three-day crash course in Vipassana meditation and the campus "sitting club" around the same time I signed up for psychology classes—simply out of curiosity about myself. Meditation is not always a formal practice in my life, but the mental flexibility of being able to turn my focus has served me well.

These days I like to start my day, when I can, sitting with a blanket around me, facing east. Yoga also helps still my thoughts. There are so many ways to practice mindfulness. Go with what works for you. Whether guided by an app, in silence, or to music, thinking about your breath, looking at a candle, or saying a mantra, it's all good. Turn to "Finding Micromoments" on page 92 for a foolproof way to get started.

Another key element of mindfulness is releasing judgment, especially self-judgment. Can you see how this could be helpful for your PPD?

Recent research has focused more narrowly on mindfulness-based cognitive therapy (MBCT), which combines a 30-minute daily mindfulness practice with some of the same cognitive behavioral therapy (CBT) tools we have been discussing. Specifically, MBCT has been shown to significantly reduce the level of depression in perinatal women. This combination of mindfulness practices and CBT can also help *prevent PPD* in women with a history of depression and help women manage the symptoms of premenstrual dysphoric disorder.

Hearing about encouraging research, do you think you would like to incorporate more mindfulness, such as meditation or yoga, into your day?

What might you do?

How do you think it could help you?

Finding Micromoments

I love self-care and mindfulness, but I also fear that self-care has become another burden on busy new parents. Do you picture spending half the day at the spa? Having childcare in place to drive to an hour-long yoga class and back? Fortunately, those are not the only options.

Sometimes, the best we can do is find micromoments of mindfulness. I look for the micromoments while sitting at a red light, before getting out of my car and transitioning between work and home, or during the brief break between clients. These moments are quick chances to reset with a few deep breaths. Here are some suggestions you might like. Put a check mark (✓) beside the ones you can *definitely* do and a star (*) beside the ones you *might* do.

_____ Take one minute to focus on your breath, connecting with your body and feeling grounded in the right here, right now.

_____ If you work, take a minute in your car when you get home before rushing into the house. Just breathe and focus on you.

_____ If you are parenting full-time and have a partner or relative, ask for a few minutes to yourself when they come home. You could mindlessly scroll social media (no judgment here!), but you will get more benefit from doing a brief guided meditation, taking a walk around the block, or doing a few yoga stretches.

_____ If you get the opportunity to go to the bathroom by yourself, maximize the experience by using your favorite soap to wash your hands. Smell the scent and give yourself a pep talk in the mirror. You've got this!

_____ Find some calm by practicing mindfulness while doing household chores. When washing the dishes, let your mind focus on the feel of the water and let other worries slip away.

_____ Try a walking meditation when pushing your baby in the stroller or when wearing a carrier. Focus on the feelings and sensations of your body moving.

Have some ideas of your own? Write them down here:

Identify at least one or two critical times in your day. For example, when do you feel most stressed?

Now make a list of a few ways you could take a micromoment.

What would your day be like if you followed through and practiced mindful moments at least once a day?

What could your life be like if it became a daily habit?

Your PPD Toolbox

Once you've had a chance to read through a bunch of the tools and strategies in this workbook, practice them, and reflect on what works for you, take some time to think about which ones will be the most helpful for you. Which tool or strategy had the biggest impact? Which is your new go-to? Which are now the Swiss army knives in your PPD toolbox?

1. _____

2. _____

3. _____

4. _____

5. _____

6. _____

7. _____

8. _____

9. _____

10. _____

11. _____

12. _____

13. _____

14. _____

15. _____

Postpartum Depression in Real Life

What does life with PPD actually look like? I've gathered some of the more common questions my clients worry about here, paired with practical advice and suggestions of things you can do in the moment to make the situation better. Please note that I would never share the private stories of any of my therapy clients. However, these are the questions that *all my clients* ask. See if any of them are issues you have wondered about, too. Feel free to jump around to any of the real-life scenarios for relevant advice, simple tips, and more CBT exercises.

Lack of Baby Bonding

It's been six weeks and I still haven't bonded with my baby. Everybody says they are "so in love" with their babies. What's wrong with me that I don't feel love for my baby?

Not every mother feels love for her baby instantly. For some, love comes much later. It is not unusual for those who have a history of trauma, a difficult birth, or serious postpartum mental health symptoms to feel less attached. Bonding might take longer, but your love can still grow.

First, don't judge yourself. If you are taking the time to read this workbook, chances are you care about your baby and how you parent. Can you reflect for a moment on how you already demonstrate love?

I'd like to point out the difference between attachment and attunement. *Attunement* refers to how well you notice your baby's needs and respond to them and is actually more important at this stage of your baby's life. Can you tell when your baby needs a diaper change or is hungry or tired? Are you able to respond appropriately? If so, take pride.

Further, for some, loving their baby is less love at first sight and more arranged marriage. Think about it: Did you select this baby from a range of choices, or is this just who you ended up with? Many adults in arranged marriages report that the relationship was awkward at first, but they eventually learned to love each other.

GROW YOUR LOVE

After reading the response above, if you would still like to increase your bonding, try singing to your baby, reading them books daily, and talking to them more. Instead of waiting to feel love, practice it first. It will come.

One of the best things you can do for your baby is to keep working on your PPD symptoms. Although depression can lower your ability to respond appropriately to your baby, research indicates CBT helps increase it. So keep working!

What are some bonding exercises you would like to try this week?

The Perfectionism Trap

I feel like I'm failing as a mom. I know some people may say I'm a perfectionist and have unrealistic standards, but I'm used to accomplishing my goals 100 percent. Now I feel like a hot mess.

When you are used to achieving and holding yourself to high standards, becoming a parent can be so hard. On the one hand, you might think the tasks of baby care are simple or easy. Yet, the hours are grueling. And remember, if this is your first child, you are still a novice.

You might have worked in your career for years. Most people need at least six months to feel comfortable at a new job. Unfortunately, once you master the skills of caring for a newborn, your baby has grown into a crawler! (See "I Miss Going to Work" on page 133 for a related discussion.)

D. W. Winnicott, an English pediatrician who helped shape the foundation of developmental psychology, taught that a "good enough" parent is the goal. Not a perfect parent. Just good enough.

Instead of striving for an A+ on your parenting report card today, would you be okay with just passing?

RATE YOURSELF

Be fair: What was your letter grade today? _____

Are you okay with that? Why or why not?

_____

_____

BATTER, BATTER, BATTER

Let's take it a step further. Baseball players measure their batting average as their number of hits divided by their number of at bats, carried to three decimal places. A batter who gets 3 hits out of 10 at bats has a batting average of .300. "Batting 300" in Major League Baseball is very good. High-level professional athletes have trained full time for years in their sport. You might still be a parenting rookie.

What was your batting average today? _____
Still struggling? Try going back to "All-or-Nothing Mamas" on page 25 and "Challenging Automatic Negative Thoughts" on page 29.

Asking for Help Is Hard

I'm really struggling. There's just too much to do and it's just so hard. Everything I read says that I should ask for help, but I wish people would just offer so I didn't have to ask.

Looking after a baby really is hard. There truly is so much to do.

Please remember, humans are not meant to raise babies in the isolation of a nuclear family. We need a village of aunties and cousins to cook, clean, and hold the baby. (See "Mothering the Mother and Matrescence" on page 71.)

Many of us have been raised to value being self-sufficient and independent. I know I was. I'd like to introduce the idea of seasons of life. In general, you are in a productive life stage. You are strong and can work and care for those older and younger than yourself. But briefly, during the postpartum stage, you are in a season of needing more support.

Accept it. Would you be willing to help a friend with a new baby? I bet you would. Then why is it hard for you to ask for the same? Think of asking your friends for help as a gift to them. You are setting a new precedent that it is okay not to be okay and it is okay to need support. Now they will feel more comfortable doing the same.

WHAT HELP DO YOU NEED?

What can you outsource? If you don't have the financial resources to hire help, what friends and family do you have? What would be a help? For example, would you like to have a meal delivered or one morning a week to yourself? A full night's sleep? Next, brainstorm one or two people you could ask.

CURRENT NEED	SOURCE OF HELP
I'm overcooking dinner all the time.	Shonda posts great casseroles on her Instagram all the time and did say, "Tell me if you need anything." Diana has set up three mealtrains for friends—maybe she'd do one for me.
I need to get more sleep.	I can go over our budget with my in-laws to see if they can help us hire a postpartum doula three nights a week.

Postpartum Rage

More than depressed, I'm angry. I'm just pissed off all the time. The littlest of things sends me into a rage. I can see that my anger is out of proportion, but I can't stop it. I'm afraid my partner will leave if I can't control it.

I can't tell you how many clients have told me they didn't know postpartum rage was real until they had suffered for months or even years. Even those aware of PPD don't connect their anger as a potential symptom of PPD. Sadly, they consider it a personal character flaw and don't ask for help.

Postpartum anger is often directed at the adult closest to us—our partner. Just as children who behave like angels at preschool will morph into monsters for their parents, adults will unconsciously feel like it is safe to be their worst in front of their closest support. Unfortunately, this tendency takes a toll on relationships.

Many times, female-identifying people will judge themselves for feeling angry. And the guilt that follows just confounds the picture.

WRITE IT OUT

Your own personal relationship with anger is likely complicated. Take some time to write about how you were raised to deal with or express anger. Was anger allowed?

How freely do you express your anger? For example, do you stuff it or ignore it until it explodes? Do you think it's important to respond to everything that annoys you?

Do you think your communication about anger is working for you and your relationship currently?

For more help, see "Postpartum Anger" on page 46 and the free downloadable anger workbook in the Resources section at the back of this workbook.

I Feel Broken

I had a traumatic birth experience and pregnancy, and now I just feel like I'm broken. I'm damaged goods. I don't think I'll ever be the same.

After any profound experience, it's unlikely that you will ever be the same as before. Similarly, after you have been pregnant and had a child, you are forever changed. But I do have hope you will one day be okay with who you have become.

Have you ever seen the Japanese pottery style called *kintsugi*?

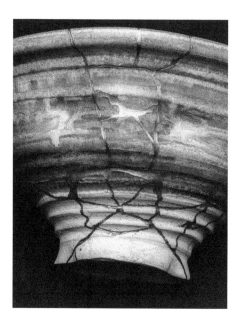

Kintsugi means "golden joinery." Broken or cracked plates, bowls, and vases are not discarded. Instead, they are carefully put back together, the pieces mended with a resin mixed with powdered gold or silver. The seams are strikingly visible in the finished piece and enhance its beauty, and the cracks and repairs become part of the piece's history.

I believe we can grow as a result of trauma, perhaps more than we ever would have grown had it not occurred.

I am sorry for what happened to you. Perinatal trauma and loss may leave you literally and emotionally ripped apart. Please know you are not damaged goods. You are beautiful, worthy, and whole. Your experiences are a part of your story.

Please visit the section "Yes, And . . . " on page 42 to read more about having a dual awareness of both the trauma and being okay right now. For example, "*Yes*, this is hard, *and* I can do hard things."

One day you will be able to complete the sentence, "Yes, this happened, and . . . "

Many people mistakenly try to console grief and trauma by pushing for meaning or a silver lining. It is more than okay if you aren't ready to see a silver (or gold) lining yet. Or ever. You can take all the time you need to grieve and feel sad. However, if you feel like you might be ready to take a stab at looking at your experiences from a side that may be more helpful for you, use the space under "This Happened" below.

THIS HAPPENED

Write about what happened. For example, what about your pregnancy, the birth, or your postpartum experience went or has gone wrong?

AND . . .

Write about how you are growing and thriving now. If you aren't able to see this part yet, do you have a trusted friend or therapist who can help you reflect in this way?

_____

_____

_____

_____

_____

_____

_____

This is hard work. After pushing yourself in your growth, whether it is through writing or simply reading these steps, make sure you also take time to slow down and soothe.

Past Trauma

I've done a bunch of therapy/personal growth in the past. I already made peace with my childhood. But lately, I feel like I'm dwelling on old stuff I thought I was over years ago. Why is it coming up again?

As a therapist, I have observed time and time again that overcoming trauma is a lifelong process. I love that you have grown and worked through past adverse childhood experiences. All that work was not for nothing. You will be able to draw on your resilience and the strategies that helped you in the past.

However, I do believe you will have to unpack and reprocess it again from the point of view of this new developmental life stage.

For example, if you had a complicated relationship with a parent growing up, it makes sense that you will reflect upon it differently now that you are a parent. You might know that you want to be a different kind of parent than your parents were and put a lot of pressure on yourself to do things according to your own standards. Or, perhaps, this new point of view as a parent makes you realize for the first time all the ways your parents made mistakes and failed you.

Some postpartum women are surprised by how an old sexual trauma can pop up. Obstetrical providers might unwittingly trigger reminders by touching them without asking for consent first. Other times, obstetric violence is a primary trauma, including unconsented episiotomies.

Therapy and the guided journaling we do here can help you unpack, sort through, and repack old baggage so you feel more in control of it.

Try this next exercise.

WHAT DID YOU AS A CHILD/TEEN/YOUNG ADULT NEED TO HEAR?

Write a letter to yourself at a pivotal age. Did you need unconditional love or protection? Using the wisdom and love you now have, write to yourself at age _____ (fill in the blank). What words did you most need to hear?

If you are currently in therapy, this is a good exercise to bring to your therapist. This letter can be hard to write or read aloud without a safe space and guidance.

Body Tension

I feel so tense and on edge all the time. I can't stop worrying. I feel like I just can't relax.

Feeling tense and anxious is very common for people with PMADs. Want to try an easy relaxation exercise?

RELAXING BODY SCAN

Lie down somewhere comfortable. Close your eyes. Take a deep breath in. As you breathe out, visualize the tension leaving your body.

Starting at the top of your head, scan your face for any tension. If you notice any tightness at your temples or in your jaw, let it out as you exhale.

Continue scanning your body, moving down your neck and shoulders, your arms and hands, your torso and back, and finally your legs and feet. Any time you find tension, picture it floating out of you on the exhale or flying out your fingertips or toes.

Take one more deep breath, scanning your body for any tension.

Next, just lie there, relaxed. Take a moment to notice the difference from how you felt before the exercise. Seal this feeling of relaxation into your muscle memory. You can come back to this feeling any time you want.

Who Has Time for Mindfulness?

People keep talking about mindfulness, but I don't think it's for me. I'm just not that woo-woo, and I don't have time to sit and meditate for an hour.

Guess what? Mindful meditation is not just for a certain kind of person, and even a few minutes of practice during the day can have powerful effects. Even if you have tried it and thought it wasn't for you, you might like to try an easy exercise now.

There is no right way to meditate or practice mindfulness. But here is a suggestion for how to quickly get started:

→ Find a comfortable place to sit, any fairly upright position that feels good to you.
→ Play some soft music or listen to a pleasant sound.
→ Either close your eyes or softly gaze at a flower, candle, plant, or incense.
→ Notice your breath and how it feels.
→ Keep turning your focus back to your breath.

That's it! Try it for a short amount of time, like two minutes. It will feel hard, but that's okay. Don't judge yourself if your mind doesn't focus. That is totally normal. Simply notice that your mind wandered and bring it back to your breath.

I believe it's the act of deciding and choosing to turn your focus back to your breath that matters. Therefore, don't judge yourself if you need to turn back often, as that's a good thing.

Once two minutes feels comfortable, you can try extending the observation, without judgment, to 5 or 10 minutes.

If you would like to listen to someone guiding you through this exercise, check the Resources section at the back of this workbook for a list of my favorite apps for relaxing, mindfulness, and meditation. You can also review "Mindful Meditation" on page 90 and "Finding Micromoments" on page 92.

Is Breast Always Best?

I've seen five lactation consultants, used nipple shields and an SNS*, and nursed then pumped around the clock, day and night. I still can't make enough milk for my baby. I feel like I'm failing at being a mother. I never leave the house, I feel like a cow, and I'm still literally insufficient. (*supplemental nursing system)

Oh mama, your worth is not defined by ounces. You are doing so much to give your baby the best.

Do you know what's even better than breast milk? A healthy and happy mother.

~~BREAST IS BEST~~

FED IS BEST

Any way you choose to feed your baby is caring and nourishing. And guess what? You don't have to decide today between exclusively breastfeeding, exclusively pumping, or exclusively formula feeding. I don't judge any of those paths and neither should you.

I encourage you to stop seeing the matter as an all-or-nothing choice between breast milk and formula. Check out "All-or-Nothing Mamas" on page 25. Maybe you simply drop one of the middle-of-the-night pumping sessions and then evaluate how it feels.

If you supplement one feed a day with formula, could it ease up some of the pressure? Your baby would still get the immunity benefits of *some* breast milk. Could you then enjoy breastfeeding more?

TIME TO REFLECT

How is breastfeeding going?

What "Negative Filters" (see page 25) are affecting the pressure you are putting on yourself?

What would help *you* feel better?

D-MER: I Get the Worst Feeling Nursing

I hate breastfeeding. It's strange. When I start nursing and feel the letdown, all of a sudden I'm filled with despair and panic and I feel like I want to cry. It happens every time we nurse, even when nothing is wrong. I want to wean, but I feel guilty for being selfish.

You might have dysphoric milk-ejection reflex, known as D-MER. Women with D-MER experience a sudden burst of negative feelings in the first few minutes of breastfeeding. For some people, it is mild and might not even be noticeable if they also have PPD. For others, the sensations are severe, even as extreme as thoughts of suicide.

Researchers think the response is tied to hormones. For most women, oxytocin is released during breastfeeding, causing milk ejection. This love hormone is also supposed to help you bond with your baby and create pleasure, increasing the chances of nourishing your baby and increasing your baby's survival. Unfortunately, for women with D-MER, their hormone system switches into extreme distress instead of triggering love and peace.

I'm sorry this is happening to you. It seems like a cruel trick of nature to instead activate your stress response. Read up on "Emotional Flooding (aka the Fight or Flight Response)" on page 49.

WHAT CAN I DO FOR D-MER?

Don't give up and wean right away. Breastfeeding is still beneficial to your mood and PPD, even if you have D-MER. You may ultimately wean, but try some of these strategies first:

Create Safety. If your body is going into fight or flight mode when nursing, try to set the scene for feeling safe and comfy. Surround yourself with people you trust. Make the place you nurse warm and cozy. Remind yourself that you and your baby are loved and cherished.

Skin to Skin. Resting before, during, and after nursing in a relaxed, skin-to-skin position can better ease stress for both mom and baby. For mothers, relaxing skin to skin can lower cortisol (the stress hormone), override the negative D-MER reaction, evoke calm, and increase bonding. Massaging your baby or asking your partner to massage you can also help.

Mindfulness. Visit the sections on "Mindful Meditation" (page 90) and "Who Has Time for Mindfulness?" (page 110) to learn ways to switch off the stress response and move into a relaxed state. Mindfulness, especially combined with the CBT-based exercises in this workbook, can help you regulate an overactive stress response. Focus on your breath, observe sensations without judging, and remind yourself that this moment will pass. You can also try the exercise for "Body Tension" on page 109.

Know You Are Not Alone. Visit the website D-MER.org to read more about D-MER. On the website, you will find firsthand accounts of others with D-MER, as well as more solutions to dealing with the condition than are given here.

I'm the Only One Who . . .

Sometimes I feel like I'm the only one who's losing it, who's failing at motherhood, and who doesn't have it together. I can't talk to anyone about what I'm feeling. My partner, family, and friends will just judge me. I'm totally alone.

First, let's look at the numbers. One in five women and one in ten partners have PPD. You simply aren't the only one.

Why does it not seem like it?

Sadly, at least half of depressed mothers never receive any help or services.

I'm curious, where are you seeing that everybody has it together? (My kids are school-aged, and I still don't have it together.)

If it's because of stuff you find on social media, then in the words of Postpartum Support International Trainer Birdie Meyer, "Everybody is lying." Others just aren't being real.

FIND THE REAL PEOPLE

Shame grows in secrecy. It evaporates in the light of day. Speaking the secret takes the power away from fears.

Where could you find others being real?

What would it be like for you to open up to even just one person?

What could you gain from sharing?

_____

_____

_____

_____

_____

How could your sharing benefit the other person?

_____

_____

_____

_____

_____

When It Seems Like You'll Never Get Better

Nothing is working. I'm doing everything I'm supposed to, but I'm still so depressed. I feel like I will never get better.

This is hard. I'm not arguing with you there. But I do have hope that this too shall pass.

And don't stop all your hard work on developing coping skills and healthy living. These practices might be making the difference between maintaining the level you're at now and falling into even deeper depression.

Remember that a key feature of PPD is hopelessness. Depression clouds your outlook and filters everything to seem even more dismal. When you're down, it's harder to notice the moments of happiness.

For more help, check out "Negative Filters," especially "All-or-Nothing Mamas," on page 25.

CRACKS IN THE MARBLE

I acknowledge how hard this time has been for you. And I see the possibility that it will get better.

If everything seems dark and dismal and you can't picture a sunny day, try to imagine a tiny crack of light. Maybe your day was black granite marble with one tiny line of bright quartz.

What was your one tiny moment of light today?

What you focus on grows. In time, you could grow your attention from one tiny joy to a daily gratitude practice. Could you journal three positive moments each day?

Try it now. List three small things that happened today for which you are grateful.

1. _____

2. _____

3. _____

With persistence, you can change the composition of your marble.

My Partner Doesn't Get It

My partner and I used to have an amazing relationship. She was my favorite person and always supported me. But now she just doesn't seem to get it. I can tell she's stressed out, too, but I wish she could give me more.

You are not alone. Two-thirds of couples experience less satisfaction in their relationship after the birth of a baby.

Yet, I do think you are on to something. Your partner might not be able to be your sole support right now. This is common, understandable, *and* a legitimate loss. You can take some time to grieve the loss of the connection you once had.

I am hopeful your relationship can grow in new ways.

In the meantime, I encourage you to diversify your support network. I don't believe one relationship can or should meet all your needs.

FILL UP YOUR DANCE CARD

Let's look at your different emotional and relationship needs. Think about all the connections your partner has given you over the years, as well as the new needs you have now as a new parent. (Suggestions include talking about your day, understanding breastfeeding struggles, sharing enjoyment in your baby's cuteness, listening to you vent, and going on walks with you.) List them under "Emotional Need." Next, brainstorm at least two or three potential new people or groups who could meet each of these needs. List them under "Alternate Source."

EMOTIONAL NEED	ALTERNATE SOURCE

Next, what needs do you most want your partner to meet or can't you out-source? For example, sexual and/or romantic intimacy, shared decision-making, coparenting, or a big bear hug. If you narrow down your list of needs, they could be more manageable for your partner. Write down these needs here:

Finally, don't assume your partner knows your new needs. Sit down and tell them.

Why Is Everything Out of Control?

Why does everything happen to me? First I couldn't get pregnant, then I had a horrible pregnancy and difficult birth, and now it all feels out of control.

Fertility is one of the true mysteries of the universe.

Birth is equally beyond our control, beautiful and wild.

Revisit the "Reproductive Story" sections (pages 37 to 41). Please know that your journey to becoming a mother is not a step-by-step process like other accomplishments in your life.

CONSIDER A RADICAL SHIFT IN VIEW

Would one of these practices help you find a more helpful point of view? Place a check mark beside each suggestion you might like to try.

☐ Learn about your ancestral birthing practices

☐ Create art

☐ Connect with nature

☐ Read about fertility rites and mythology

☐ Nourish your inner goddess

☐ Subvert the dominant paradigm and decolonize your bookshelf

☐ Spend time with female elders and hear their stories

☐ Learn about other cultures and their differences and similarities

☐ Journal

☐ Look for the sacred in this journey

☐ Turn to your higher power and prayer

☐ Meditate

SURF THE WAVE

Want one more tool? Imagine the ocean. We cannot control something so huge and vast. The waves and tide come and go. Do you try to hold back the waves or rising tide?

No. You watch. We cannot control the waves, but we can watch them rise and fall. We observe without judging, without fighting.

We will never control the ocean. But, in time, we may learn to surf.

A Healthy Baby Is Not All That Matters

***Birth really didn't go the way I had hoped. Everyone says all that matters is a
healthy baby, but I'm not okay with it.***

You are entitled to grieve the loss of the birth you wanted or expected.

I define a traumatic birth liberally, including any of the following. Check off those
that apply to you.

- ☐ Did not feel in control of my body

- ☐ Did not have my choices honored by the medical providers

- ☐ Perceived fear of losing the baby

- ☐ Perceived fear of serious injury or issue with the baby

- ☐ Perceived fear of my own life being in danger

- ☐ Did not feel empowered in my choices

- ☐ Felt the birth did not go as expected

Yes, you have a living baby, and you are struggling with the birth. Both truths are
important to acknowledge.

For more work on this, write out your birth story using "Your Reproductive Story"
(page 37) and "Your Story Continues" (page 41).

In time, you can use dual awareness, discussed in "Yes, And . . ." (page 42), to see
both the beauty and the brutality of the birth experience.

Stillbirth

I delivered a stillborn baby last month. Can I have PPD if I don't have a live baby?

First, I am so, so sorry. You have gone through all the pain and suffering of childbirth and have been left with the worst possible outcome.

Sixty to 70 percent of mothers grieving a stillbirth experience depressive symptoms one year later. Fifty percent have symptoms for four years or more. Clearly, we don't just get over it.

WHAT HELPS AFTER A STILLBIRTH, A MISCARRIAGE, OR INFANT LOSS?

Compassion. During and immediately after a stillbirth, having respectful and compassionate medical providers can make a difference. Have compassion for yourself as you honor your baby. Your pregnancy and child mattered and still matter.

Mementos. If you have any physical mementos or photographs of your lost baby, treasure them. Some parents keep their baby's hospital bracelet and photos but do not display them. They may feel embarrassed to share them. I encourage families to be proud of the little one who was and remains a special part of their family. If you do not have any mementos, consider buying a special candle or planting something in your garden as a physical reminder.

Rituals. Perinatal loss is a disenfranchised loss, meaning that we feel alone and lost about how to mark the passing. As much as possible, try to practice rituals to mark your baby's life. Perhaps you can make a small altar and light a special candle.

Meaning. Grief is a heart opener. I wouldn't wish it on anyone, but now that you have experienced it, one day you may even appreciate its gifts. One friend of mine started a random acts of kindness campaign in honor of her stillborn daughter.

Resources. Turn back to the sections related to the reproductive story (starting on page 37). Look up the Star Legacy Foundation and others in the Resources section.

Pregnancy After Loss

I'm pregnant again after a miscarriage. I'm thrilled and hopeful, but I'm also worried it will happen again. I'm sad that I'm not enjoying this pregnancy. When we went in for the ultrasound, instead of being happy and excited, I was filled with dread. It just reminds me of when we learned there was no heartbeat last time.

Congratulations on your pregnancy! And welcome to the anxious world of pregnancy after loss. Of course you have fears after such a traumatic experience. How could you not?

Our challenge now is to balance the dueling emotions. Many parents are surprised to find that they don't feel "all better" or "fixed" once they are pregnant again after a miscarriage, stillbirth, or termination for medical reasons. Please don't judge yourself if you find this harder than you expected. I believe you can find courage and hope while honoring all your babies and your grief journey.

WHAT STAGE OF PREGNANCY AFTER LOSS ARE YOU IN?

Dr. Joann O'Leary of the Star Legacy Foundation writes about the "the developmental tasks" of pregnancy after loss. Review each stage of pregnancy below and its associated characteristics. Place a check mark next to the tasks you are currently working on.

PRECONCEPTION

☐ Deciding to try again

☐ Finding hope

☐ Not being in sync with my partner

☐ Feeling empty and needing a baby

☐ Feeling like a failure

FIRST TRIMESTER

☐ Excitement plus panic

☐ Being aware of every ache and pain

☐ Desperate to see the heartbeat

- ☐ My partner is scared to touch me
- ☐ Not wanting to talk about the new baby
- ☐ Scared and happy at the same time

SECOND TRIMESTER

- ☐ Fear of losing the baby
- ☐ Surprise that the pregnancy hasn't made me feel better
- ☐ PTSD
- ☐ Worry I'm being disloyal to the baby who died
- ☐ Conflicted about announcing the pregnancy
- ☐ My partner is weird and ambivalent

24 TO 32 WEEKS GESTATION

- ☐ Wanting to rush through this stage
- ☐ Decreased anxiety as weeks pass and viability increases
- ☐ Turning inward
- ☐ Worry that anxiety might cause contractions
- ☐ My partner feels left out and hopeless

32 WEEKS TO BIRTH

- ☐ It finally feels real—I'm going to have a baby
- ☐ I feel more grief over my lost baby

BIRTH

☐ Not feeling joy but some relief

☐ There is a new layer of grief

☐ I'm worried the baby will die

☐ I feel guilty enjoying this baby

☐ My partner is now falling apart

Pregnancy after loss is very hard. If you had been on the fence about starting therapy or joining a support group, and you checked off more than a couple of the tasks and/or issues above, please consider finding more support. Visit the Resources section for groups that support families after a loss (page 149) and for suggestions about how to find a therapist who specializes in perinatal loss.

Rainbow Babies Aren't All Sunshine

After my share of storms, I finally have my rainbow baby. I thought I would be happy now, but I'm not. I'm just not enjoying it as much as I thought I would and that makes me feel ungrateful and guilty.

Many who suffer a pregnancy loss dream of the day they will be able to hold a live baby. Some call the baby born after such a storm their "rainbow" baby.

Sometimes, the goal of a live birth is seen as the end goal for so long that, once you get there, you haven't much planned for how you will feel afterward.

A rainbow baby doesn't fix everything. Sometimes that realization alone is a colossal letdown.

Others feel gratitude for their new baby, but do not enjoy every minute. This is normal. This is healthy. Having a new baby is hard. Please don't judge yourself if it isn't rainbows and unicorns all the time.

Having had a previous loss puts you at an increased risk of PPD as well as postpartum anxieties, including postpartum PTSD and OCD. Doesn't that make sense, though? After the worst has happened (losing a child), it's completely understandable that you would be fearful and vigilant of something happening again.

Please don't judge yourself. Visit "Negative Filters" (page 25), "Challenging Automatic Negative Thoughts" (page 29), "Mindful Meditation" (page 90), and "Yes, And . . ." (page 42) for more tools.

Recovery and Wine Mom Culture

I struggled with alcohol when I was younger, but I have been sober for five years. I don't connect with a lot of mom groups and have a hard time with all the joking about wine and wine moms.

First, happy five years! Your recovery is a huge accomplishment and you should be proud.

I don't believe your discomfort is unreasonable. Over the past decade, problem drinking, or drinking so much it causes problems in one's life, rose 83 percent in women. High-risk alcohol use, or having four or more drinks in a day, rose 58 percent in women.

Simultaneously, the theme of "wine moms" became popular in social media memes, television, and movies. It's hard not to make a connection. Unfortunately, popular culture is sending out a message that moms drinking to cope is funny and cute.

Remember, you don't need to drink to get through parenting. On the flip side, your recovery skills are going to help you with your PPD.

MY RECOVERY TOOLS

You can now draw on all the things that worked for you getting sober. Regardless of whether or not you are struggling in your sobriety, the same tools can help you with living life on life's terms. Check off the tools you have used in the past and/or might want to try now.

I want to try . . .

- ☐ Taking it "one day at a time"
- ☐ Not getting too hungry, angry, lonely, or tired (HALT)
- ☐ Going back to meetings
- ☐ Saying the Serenity Prayer
- ☐ Reconnecting with my sponsor
- ☐ Remembering "this too shall pass"
- ☐ Calling other moms and sober friends
- ☐ Reading recovery books

- ☐ Drawing on my higher power
- ☐ Using my mindfulness tools
- ☐ Pausing before reacting
- ☐ Doing step work around PPD or a birth topic
- ☐ Finding nondrinking mom friends
- ☐ *Add your own:* _____

Body Image Issues

I've never had a great relationship with how my body looks, but my post-baby weight is making me really unhappy. It doesn't help that everyone I follow on social media looks amazing, thin, and happy in their posts.

Ah, comparison is the thief of joy.

Most of my clients know better than to compare their real life to someone else's highlight reel. They know social media is, literally and figuratively, a filtered selection. But even if we know people only post their most put-together images on Facebook, why do we compare these photos to our day-to-day chaos?

If you had a C-section, had diastasis recti, are over the age of 30, or had a larger frame pre-baby, it may take longer than nine months to take the weight off. Some bodies hold on to fat to help with milk production. You may understand rationally that you won't look like a 22-year-old model post-baby. Yet, you may find yourself unfavorably comparing your body with theirs.

Social comparison theory explains that we look at others around us and compare how we rate in order to understand ourselves. Unfortunately, the most commonly experienced emotions felt when scrolling Instagram and Facebook are envy and shame.

CURATE YOUR FEED

Many of us find ourselves mindlessly scrolling social media. When you are brain-dead and nursing or rocking in the middle of the night, it seems like an easy distraction.

I'd like you to start to notice how your social media feed makes you feel. You might want to limit your social media consumption.

Better yet, be intentional about what accounts you follow. This is your official permission to stop following or mute the people who make you feel bad about yourself. Research shows that when social media no longer evokes your envy, depression can lessen.

Indeed, social media can actually be a wonderful source of support. Therapists are now sharing nuggets of advice on Instagram. (I myself focus on quick tips for postpartum mental health @burdtherapy.) You can find a list of Instagram accounts and hashtags to follow in the Resources section.

You might like to find others celebrating body positivity and being real about both the beauty and the brutality of postpartum life. If your feed is celebrating what your body can *do* as opposed to how it looks, it will be easier for you to do the same. See also "Postpartum Body Image" on page 53.

NOTE: If you have a history of an eating disorder, please consider seeking out extra support. Eating disorders are often overlooked and underdiagnosed during pregnancy and postpartum. Yet such a disorder is understandably triggered to flare up. If your usual tools for keeping a healthy relationship to food and your body aren't working, consider getting back into treatment.

I Miss Going to Work

Maybe I'm not meant to be a mother. This is both hard and boring. I miss going to work. I was better at my job than I am at this.

You are not alone in missing work, whether you are on a brief maternity leave or taking longer to be home with your child(ren). Take some time to acknowledge that you are truly experiencing loss. It is possible to want to provide this time to your baby *and* suffer as a result.

LOSSES DURING MATERNITY

Circle the losses you have experienced as a result of the transition to motherhood.

Community   Socializing   Control

Previous Self   Peace of Mind

Intimacy

Independence   Adult Conversations

Spontaneity

Identity   Predictability   Quiet

Hobbies   Relationships   Money

Sleep   Accomplishment   Friends

Self-Confidence   Purpose   "Me" Time

Professional Growth   Feeling Experienced

Intellectual Stimulation   Career

What else have you lost as a result of not working and transitioning to parenting?

_____

_____

_____

_____

Remember, you are new at this. You will gain more experience and settle in over time. Visit "The Perfectionism Trap" on page 99 for a related discussion.

Take time to grieve the loss of the person you once were, and take time to ultimately like the person you have become.

I Feel Guilty About Not Contributing Financially

My partner and I are okay financially without me working, but I feel guilty for not contributing. Because I don't work, I have been getting up every night with the baby every time he wakes. Chronic sleep deprivation is getting to me, but I don't feel entitled to ask for help because I don't have to go to work.

Guess what? You are on the job. It's just that instead of working 40 hours in a week, you are on the clock 24/7. Stay-at-home parents work, on average, the equivalent of 2.5 full-time jobs, or 100 hours a week.

Frankly, being well rested is vital to your baby's safety, as well as crucial to your ability to manage the symptoms of PMADs. See "How to Communicate Your Needs" (page 66) for tips on respecting and discussing your needs and your partner's.

Further, you are likely underestimating your current financial contribution to the family. In a household with both partners working outside the home and no children, it is easier to see the value of each partner's financial input. However, research shows that women in heterosexual relationships who work outside the home are more likely to still do a larger share of household chores and the invisible "mental load."

Women in heterosexual relationships are more likely to be the default parent who keeps track of the doctor's visits, writes the thank-you notes, and assumes the kinship responsibilities for both sides of the family. Other examples of invisible labor include keeping the calendar, planning parties and trips, and taking on responsibility for the emotional welfare of everyone in the family.

If you are not earning a paycheck from an external source, you may not appreciate the full savings you bring to the family. Without your full-time parenting, what duties would you have to outsource and pay someone else to do?

STAY-AT-HOME PAYCHECK CALCULATOR

At the time of this writing, Salary.com calculates the median value of the work of a full-time parent to be equivalent to an annual salary of US$162,581. You can personalize the calculation with your duties and location on their website.

In the following table, check off the jobs you do and estimate how many hours per week you spend doing them.

Are you still feeling guilty about not contributing financially? Maybe not so much, right?

√	JOB TITLE	TYPICAL HOURS PER WEEK
	Childcare Provider	
	Cook	
	Wet Nurse	
	Laundry Machine Operator	
	Housekeeper	
	Driver	
	Nutritionist	
	Logistics Analyst	
	Psychologist	
	Facilities Manager	
	CEO	
	Groundskeeper	
	Janitor	
	Plumber	
	Personal Assistant	

√	JOB TITLE	TYPICAL HOURS PER WEEK
	Travel Agent	
	Event Planner	
	Bookkeeper	
	Interior Designer	
	Computer Operator	
	Teacher	
	Spiritual Advisor	

I Worry About Going Back to Work

My paid family leave is ending soon, and I'm dreading going back to work. I don't feel good about our childcare options and my baby doesn't take a bottle.

Going back to work is a major source of anxiety and worry for new parents. If you live in a country with very limited family leave, such as the United States, you will likely feel forced to go back to work before you are ready.

WHAT'S MOST STRESSING YOU?

Anxiety bouncing around your head at night, keeping you from sleeping, doesn't help. However, good anxiety can be channeled into action. Start addressing your concerns with research and planning.

Some of the most common—and completely valid—concerns about going back to work include the following:

Childcare
Suggestions:

→ Research childcare options ahead of time.
→ Have a Plan A, Plan B, Plan C, and Plan D for when something falls through or someone cancels because of illness.
→ Talk to friends for referrals and tour childcare facilities.
→ Trust your gut when touring or interviewing a prospective childcare provider. If you don't like someone initially, it likely won't get better.
→ If you are having family watch your baby, you might be trading financial savings for control. Have a frank conversation with your family member about your expectations and about them following your wishes.

Breastfeeding and Pumping
Suggestions:

→ Take a course or read up on going back to work.
→ Start pumping once a day to build up a stash of milk.
→ Introduce a bottle ideally around one month (or as directed by a lactation consultant).
→ Have your partner or someone else give a bottle at least once a week (go out and do some self-care!) during your leave so your baby stays familiar with it.

→ Talk with your manager about what space and scheduling will be available to you for pumping.

→ Don't expect to get work done when pumping. You might find your brain is only capable of mindless tasks like deleting e-mails during this time. Try relaxing instead.

Lack of Family-Friendly Policies
Suggestions:

→ Research your rights and options for replacement income under family leave and pregnancy disability. Talk to your human resources department, and research state or government options.

→ Talk to your manager and/or union about the company's pumping policy.

→ Research your local government's policies around pumping.

→ If your PPD and anxiety will impact your ability to function at work, talk to your doctor about short-term disability for PPD.

The first day you go back to work you might cry as much as your baby. Be gentle with yourself. Remember that this transition is probably harder on you than on your baby. Trust that your baby is in good hands—you did your due diligence researching your childcare.

Good to Go!

How will I know when I'm good to go? How will I know I'm over my PPD and able to be on my own without therapy or this workbook?

You have done some amazing work so far. In what ways have your symptoms of PPD changed? Read these statements and check the ones that apply to you.

☐ I no longer feel so overwhelmed.

☐ I no longer feel as alone.

☐ I understand that there was nothing I did to cause PPD.

☐ I understand I am not to blame.

☐ I am more confident in my ability to parent.

☐ I am more comfortable asking for help.

☐ I know more ways to manage my PPD symptoms.

☐ I have more skills for managing my negative thoughts.

☐ I have more tools for self-care.

☐ I have more hope that I will feel better.

What work do you still have left to do?

_____

_____

_____

_____

SELF-ASSESS: GOOD TO GO

Here is a simple way to assess yourself moving forward. You can do this exercise on your own, once a week or daily, or make plans to check in with someone else regularly.

Picture a traffic light with three colored lights.

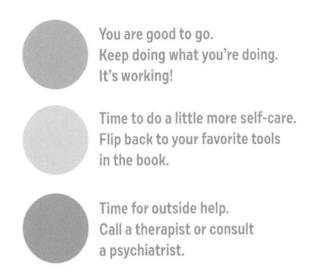

You are good to go.
Keep doing what you're doing.
It's working!

Time to do a little more self-care.
Flip back to your favorite tools
in the book.

Time for outside help.
Call a therapist or consult
a psychiatrist.

That's not so complicated, is it? Can you tell which color you are today?

Remember, You Are Not Alone

You are doing a beautiful job navigating difficult and complicated stuff. This is hard, **and** you can overcome hard things.

After finishing this workbook, I hope you will truly believe the following:

You Are Not Alone

Sometimes it feels like you are the only one home, alone and struggling. But you are not. If it seems like everyone on social media is happy and has it together, they are either lying or just showing you their best moments. (It might simply be time to change who you follow.)

Don't forget that one in five women experience PPD. Sadly, it might not seem that common because up to 85 percent of women with perinatal mood and anxiety disorders don't receive proper treatment. Give yourself a pat on the back for starting your journey here.

You Are Not to Blame

There is nothing you did to cause or create PPD. You are not to blame for any complications in your pregnancy or birth or for your child's special needs. Breastfeeding challenges are not your fault.

Perinatal depression is not a personal failure. If anything, I see it as a societal failure to support new families.

You Don't Have to Suffer

You don't deserve to be depressed. You deserve help and support.

Many of us were raised in families and cultures that celebrated the trope of the mother as martyr. Latinx cultures may limit parents of all genders with *marianismo*. Historically, many female-identified Black, Indigenous, and people of color were dehumanized and burdened with the praise of being as strong as steel, doing it all on their own.

Mothers have long been praised for being superwomen. I question the burden these images place on new mothers. I don't believe it is sustainable to place your needs last. Healthy societies need healthy families with healthy, happy mothers.

Breaking the cycles of intergenerational trauma feels like yet another burden and barrier. But I believe you can do it, aided by asking for help.

Things Can Get Better

PPD is highly treatable. If you liked the approach of this workbook, you can find a therapist who specializes in perinatal mental health and CBT in the directories listed in the Resources section.

Perhaps you are already starting to feel better. Savor the positive changes.

You've got this!

RESOURCES

Suicide Prevention Resources

In the United States, the National Suicide Prevention Lifeline is 1-800-273-8255, or call 911. The crisis text line is available 24/7 in the United States and Canada (text 741741), the UK (text 85258), and Ireland (text 086 1800 280). Other countries' hotlines are listed on SuicideStop.com.

Postpartum Support International (PSI)

Visit Postpartum.net for education on PMADs, for online support groups happening daily, and to find a local resource coordinator in your area. You can also reach out by phone and a trained volunteer will return your call or text. Call 1-800-944-4773 (4PPD) (English and Spanish), or text 503-894-9453 (English) or 971-420-0294 (Spanish).

Next, the PSI Provider Directory, PSIDirectory.com, is a great way to find therapists, psychiatrists, and therapy groups. You can search by your location, health insurance, etc. A provider with the initials "PMH-C" after their name has demonstrated their experience, training, and knowledge by exam.

Expert Medication Advice

PSI Providers line

If your primary care doctor, OB-GYN, nurse practitioner, or psychiatrist is less experienced with perinatal mental health, you can have them call the PSI Perinatal Psychiatric Consult Line at 1-800-944-4773, extension 4.

Massachusetts General Hospital (MGH) Center for Women's Mental Health

Another great resource for your medication prescriber, including the National Pregnancy Registry for Psychiatric Medication. Visit WomensMentalHealth.org.

Resources Specifically for Mothers Who Are Black, Indigenous, and People of Color

Given the structural and systemic disparities for Black mothers and other mothers who are disproportionately impacted by PPD, the following organizations are dedicated to raising awareness and creating support.

Shades of Blue Project
ShadesofBlueProject.org
@shadesofblueproject

Black Mamas Matter Alliance
BlackMamasMatter.org
@blackmamasmatter

Every Mother Counts
EveryMotherCounts.org
@everymomcounts

The Black Doula
TheBlackDoula.com
@theblackdoula

National Birth Equity Collaboration
BirthEquity.org
@birthequity

Black Emotional Mental Health Collective (BEAM)
BEAM.Community
@_beamorg

Sisters in Loss
SistersInLoss.com
@sistersinloss

Broken Brown Egg
TheBrokenBrownEgg.org
@brokenbrownegg

The Lactation Therapist
TheLactationTherapist.com
@thelactationtherapist

Shivonne Odom, LCPC, LPC, NCC, CSC
AkomaCounselingConcepts.com
@akoma_counseling

Perinatal Loss Resources

Star Legacy Foundation
Star Legacy Foundation provides live, interactive, online support groups for families who have experienced a perinatal loss and for individuals experiencing a pregnancy after a loss.
StarLegacyFoundation.org
@starlegacyfoundation

Miscarriage Hurts
A service of Life Perspectives, MiscarriageHurts.com offers many resources. The group also offers excellent training to providers.
MiscarriageHurts.com

Return to Zero: H.O.P.E.
RTZ HOPE is dedicated to "transforming the culture of silence and isolation around pregnancy and infant loss." The organization has specialized support for grieving Black and LGTBQIA parents.
RTZHope.org
@rtzhope

Books

For a frequently updated list of recommended books with links, visit BurdTherapy.com/books. Here are a few suggested titles:

The Motherly Guide to Becoming Mama: Redefining the Pregnancy, Birth, and Postpartum Journey by Jill Koziol, Liz Tenety, and Diana Spalding

The Fourth Trimester: A Postpartum Guide to Healing Your Body, Balancing Your Emotions, and Restoring Your Vitality by Kimberly Ann Johnson

The Postpartum Husband: Practical Solutions for Living with Postpartum Depression by Karen Kleiman

Good Moms Have Scary Thoughts: A Healing Guide to the Secret Fears of New Mothers by Karen Kleiman

Breathe, Mama, Breathe: 5-Minute Mindfulness for Busy Moms by Shonda Moralis

Parental Mental Health: Factoring in Fathers by Jane Honikman and Daniel B. Singley

Resources for Anger

My favorite resource for anger management is a CBT-based workbook that is free to download from the U.S. Department of Health and Human Services, Substance Abuse and Mental Health Services Administration (SAMHSA). Although the title of the workbook indicates that it was developed for people overcoming substance abuse and mental health struggles, I find the material to be relevant for anyone wanting more tools to manage their anger.

You can download *Anger Management for Substance Use Disorder and Mental Health Clients: Participant Workbook* at Store.SAMHSA.gov/product/Anger-Management -for-Substance-Use-Disorder-and-Mental-Health-Clients-Participant-Workbook /PEP19-02-01-002.

Resources for Partners and Dads

Remember, 1 in 10 men experiences postpartum depression. LGBTQIA partners are at an even higher risk of PPD. Here are some useful resources:

QueeringParenthood.com offers resources and research for LGBTQ families and those who want to support them.

PostpartumMen.com focuses on supporting men overcoming their own PPD.

Postpartum Support International hosts a free monthly "dads chat with an expert": Postpartum.net/get-help/resources-for-fathers.

Dr. Daniel B. Singley of the Center for Men's Excellence and "Basic Training for New Dads" classes has many father-focused resources on MenExcel.com.

Daddit, a subreddit, focuses on the experience of fathering in general, but mental health is discussed openly: Reddit.com/r/daddit.

Postpartum Planning and PPD Prevention

My "Prevent Postpartum Depression" Course

In 2019, I created a self-paced online course with readings, guided journaling, a private community, and short (5- to 15-minute) educational videos. Like this workbook, the emphasis of the course is on practical skills and strategies to create solutions. You can learn more at PreventPPD.com. (A second course of mine, RelationshipsAfterBaby .com, goes deeper into how you can improve your relationship with your partner.)

Postpartum Plans

Postpartum Support Virginia has a free 11-page postpartum plan you can complete that covers the following topics: rest, meals, infant feeding, older siblings, renewing and recharging, finding friends, mental health, and returning to normal. You can download the plan here: PostpartumVA.org/wp-content/uploads/2013/11/The -Postpartum-Plan.pdf.

PostpartumTogether.com offers online support, including group coaching and postpartum planning, information, and resources.

Helpful Instagram Profiles

Accounts that focus on PPD and maternal mental health:

@burdtherapy

Full disclosure: This is my professional account, but I hope the material here will support the work you have done in this workbook. I also share my latest recommended accounts to follow.

@postpartumstress (and the hashtag #SpeakTheSecret)

@fourthtrimestercollective

@momandmind (and her podcast *Mom & Mind*)

@shadesofblueproject

@postpartumsupportinternational

@postpartumhealthalliance

@mommyandme.therapist

@nayeli_lcsw

@momdocpsychology

@_happyasamother

Accounts that support new moms and parents:

@mother.ly (and their website Mother.ly)

@chels.keeps.it.real

@firstlatch

@iamksealsallers

@blackmamasmatter

@drsterlingobgyn

@imomsohard

@sobermomtribe

For transgestational, genderqueer, and non-binary parents:

@biffandi

@familyequality

For general mental health:

@makedaisychains (and the hashtag #BoringSelfCare)

@lovesomedove

@blessthemessy

@wonder_doodles

Mindfulness Apps

Expectful (perinatal focus)

Mindset

Calm

Insight Timer

Headspace

Breathe

REFERENCES

Abelsohn, Kira A., Rachel Epstein, and Lori E. Ross. "Celebrating the 'Other' Parent: Mental Health and Wellness of Expecting Lesbian, Bisexual, and Queer Non-Birth Parents," *Journal of Gay & Lesbian Mental Health* 17, no. 4 (2013): 387–405. doi: 10.1080/19359705.2013.771808.

Alhusen, Jeanne L., Kelly M. Bower, Elizabeth Epstein, and Phyllis Sharps. "Racial Discrimination and Adverse Birth Outcomes: An Integrative Review." *Journal of Midwifery & Women's Health* 61, no. 6 (2016): 707–720. doi: 10.1111/jmwh.12490.

American Psychiatric Association. *Diagnostic and Statistical Manual of Mental Disorders*, 5th ed. Washington, DC: American Psychiatric Publishing, Inc., 2013.

Bayrampour, Hamideh, Arunima Kapoor, Mary Bunka, and Deirdre Ryan. "The Risk of Relapse of Depression During Pregnancy after Discontinuation of Antidepressants," *The Journal of Clinical Psychiatry* 81, no. 4 (2020): 19r13134. doi: 10.4088/jcp.19r13134.

Beck, Aaron T., "The Past and Future of Cognitive Therapy," *The Journal of Psychotherapy and Research* 6, no. 4 (1997): 276–284.

Burd, Abigail. "Some GRAPES a Day Keep the Psychiatrist Away: A Self-Care Checklist," *Burd Psychotherapy*, August 23, 2014. BurdTherapy.com/some-grapes-a-day-keep-the-psychiatrist-away/. Accessed April 19, 2020.

———. "Prevent Postpartum Depression" (online course), 2019. PreventPPD.com.

———. "Relationships after Baby" (online course), 2020. RelationshipsAfterBaby.com.

Burns, David D. *Feeling Good: The New Mood Therapy*. New York: Morrow, 1980.

Cann, Arnie, et al., "The Core Beliefs Inventory: A Brief Measure of Disruption in the Assumptive World," *Anxiety, Stress & Coping* 23, no. 1 (2010): 19–34. doi: 10.1080/10615800802573013.

Cohen, Lee S., et al., "Relapse of Major Depression during Pregnancy in Women Who Maintain or Discontinue Antidepressant Treatment," *JAMA* 295, no. 5 (2006): 499–507. doi: 10.1001/jama.295.5.499.

Cox, John, and Jeni Holden. *Perinatal Mental Health: A Guide to the Edinburgh Postnatal Depression Scale (EPDS)*. London: Royal College of Psychiatrists, 2003.

Cox, J. L., J. M. Holden, and R. Sagovsky, "Detection of Postnatal Depression: Development of the 10-Item Edinburgh Postnatal Depression Scale," *The British Journal of Psychiatry* 150, no. 6 (1987): 782–786.

Davalos, D. B., C. A. Yadon, and H. C. Tregellas, "Untreated Prenatal Maternal Depression and the Potential Risks to Offspring: A Review," *Archive of Women's Mental Health* 15, no. 1 (2012): 1–14.

Dimidjian, Sona, et al. "An Open Trial of Mindfulness-based Cognitive Therapy for the Prevention of Perinatal Depressive Relapse/Recurrence," *Archives of Women's Mental Health* 18, no. 1 (2014): 85-94. doi: 10.1007/s00737-014-0468-x.

Dimidjian, Sona, et al., "Staying Well during Pregnancy and the Postpartum: A Pilot Randomized Trial of Mindfulness-based Cognitive Therapy for the Prevention of Depressive Relapse/Recurrence," *Journal of Consulting and Clinical Psychology* 84, no. 2 (2016): 134–145. doi: 10.1037/ccp0000068.

Dunn, Jancee. *How Not to Hate Your Husband after Kids*. London: Random House UK, 2018.

Earls, Marian F., and Committee on Psychosocial Aspects of Child and Family Health, American Academy of Pediatrics, "Incorporating Recognition and Management of Perinatal and Postpartum Depression into Pediatric Practice," *Pediatrics* 126, no. 5 (2010): 1032–1039.

Ertel, Karen A., Janet W. Rich-Edwards, and Karestan C. Koenen, "Maternal Depression in the United States: Nationally Representative Rates and Risks," *Journal of Women's Health* 20, no. 11 (2011): 1609–1617. doi: 10.1089/jwh.2010.2657.

Fidaleo, Raymond, et al. *Cognitive Therapy Manual*. San Diego, CA: Sharp Mesa Vista Hospital, Cognitive Intensive Outpatient Program, 2014.

Flanders, Corey E., Margaret F. Gibson, Abbie E. Goldberg, and Lori E. Ross, "Postpartum Depression among Visible and Invisible Sexual Minority Women: A Pilot Study," *Archives of Women's Mental Health* 19, no. 2 (2015), 299–305. doi: 10.1007/s00737-015-0566-4.

Gottman, John M., and Julie Schwartz Gottman. *And Baby Makes Three: The Six-Step Plan for Preserving Marital Intimacy and Rekindling Romance after Baby Arrives*. New York: Three Rivers Press, 2008.

Gottman, John, and Nan Silver. *Why Marriages Succeed or Fail*. London: Bloomsbury Paperbacks, 2014.

Grant, Bridget F., et al., "Prevalence of 12-Month Alcohol Use, High-Risk Drinking, and DSM-IV Alcohol Use Disorder in the United States, 2001–2002 to 2012–2013: Results from the National Epidemiologic Survey on Alcohol and Related Conditions," *JAMA Psychiatry* 74, no. 9 (2017): 911–923. doi: 10.1001/jamapsychiatry .2017.2161.

Green, Sheryl M., Erika Haber, Benicio N. Frey, and Randi E. Mccabe, "Cognitive-Behavioral Group Treatment for Perinatal Anxiety: A Pilot Study," *Archives of Women's Mental Health* 18, no. 4 (2015): 631–638. doi: 10.1007/s00737-015-0498-z.

Hoffman, Casey, Dena M. Dunn, and Wanjiku F. M. Njoroge, "Impact of Postpartum Mental Illness upon Infant Development," *Current Psychiatry Reports* 19 (2017): 100. doi: 10.1007/s11920-017-0857-8.

Huang, Lili, Yunzhi Zhao, Chunfang Qiang, and Bozhen Fan, "Is Cognitive Behavioral Therapy a Better Choice for Women with Postnatal Depression? A Systematic Review and Meta-analysis," PLoS One 13, no. 10 (2018): e0205243. doi: 10.1371/journal.pone.0205243.

Jaffe, Janet, "The Reproductive Story: Dealing with Miscarriage, Stillbirth, or Other Perinatal Demise," in *Women's Reproductive Mental Health across the Lifespan*, ed. D. L. Barnes (Springer International Publishing, 2014), 159–176. doi: 10.1007/978-3-319-05116-1_9.

Jaffe, Janet, "Trauma and the Reproductive Story," Psychotherapy.net, accessed April 19, 2020. Psychotherapy.net/article/grief/trauma-and-the-reproductive-story.

Jaffe, Janet, and Martha O. Diamond. *Reproductive Trauma: Psychotherapy with Infertility and Pregnancy Loss Clients*. Washington, DC: American Psychological Association, 2011.

Jannati, Nazanin, Shahrzad Mazhari, Leila Ahmadian, and Moghaddameh Mirzaee, "Effectiveness of an App-based Cognitive Behavioral Therapy Program for Postpartum Depression in Primary Care: A Randomized Controlled Trial," *International Journal of Medical Informatics* 141 (2020): 104145. doi: 10.1016/j.ijmedinf.2020.104145.

Keefe, Robert H., Carol Brownstein-Evans, and Rebecca S. Rouland Polmanteer, "Having Our Say: African-American and Latina Mothers Provide Recommendations to Health and Mental Health Providers Working with New Mothers Living with Postpartum Depression," *Social Work in Mental Health* 14, no. 5 (2016): 497–508. doi: 10.1080/15332985.2016.1140699.

Kleiman, Karen. *What Am I Thinking? Having a Baby after Postpartum Depression*. Bloomington, IN: Xlibris Corporation, 2005.

Kleiman, Karen R., and Molly McIntyre. *Good Moms Have Scary Thoughts: A Healing Guide to the Secret Fears of Mothers*. Sanger, CA: Familius, 2019.

Koren, Gideon, and Hedvig Nordeng, "Antidepressant Use during Pregnancy: The Benefit-Risk Ratio," *American Journal of Obstetrics and Gynecology* 207, no. 3 (2012): 157–163. doi: 10.1016/j.ajog.2012.02.009.

Kozhimannil, Katy B., et al., "Racial and Ethnic Disparities in Postpartum Depression Care among Low-Income Women, *Psychiatric Services* (Washington, DC) 62, no. 6 (2011): 619–625. doi: 10.1176/ps.62.6.pss6206_0619.

Kronenfeld, Nirit, et al., "Chronic Use of Psychotropic Medications in Breastfeeding Women: Is It Safe?" [published correction appears in PLoS One 13, no. 6 (2018): e0199906]. PLoS One 13, no. 5 (2018): e0197196. doi: 10.1371/journal.pone .0197196.

Leino, Abbie D., et al., "SSRIs in Pregnancy: What Should You Tell Your Depressed Patient?" *Current Psychiatry* 12, no. 11 (2013): 41–42, 44, accessed from MDEdge .com/psychiatry/article/78292/depression/ssris-pregnancy-what-should-you-tell -your-depressed-patient.

Lim, Myungsuh, and Yoon Yang, "Effects of Users' Envy and Shame on Social Comparison That Occurs on Social Network Services," *Computers in Human Behavior* 51, Pt. A (2015): 300–311. doi: 10.1016/j.chb.2015.05.013.

Linehan, Marsha M. *Cognitive-Behavioral Treatment of Borderline Personality Disorder*. New York: Guilford Press, 1993.

Lisitsa, Ellie, "The Four Horsemen: The Antidotes," *The Gottman Institute*, April 26, 2013. Gottman.com/blog/the-four-horsemen-the-antidotes/.

Lu, Michael C., et al., "Closing the Black-White Gap in Birth Outcomes: A Life-Course Approach," *Ethnicity & Disease* 20, 1 Suppl. 2 (2010): S2-62-76.

Luca, Dara L., et al., "Financial Toll of Untreated Perinatal Mood and Anxiety Disorders among 2017 Births in the United States," *American Journal of Public Health* 110, no. 6 (2020): 888–896. doi: 10.2105/AJPH.2020.305619.

Maccio, Elaine M., and Jaimee A. Pangburn, "The Case for Investigating Postpartum Depression among Lesbian and Bisexual Women," *Women's Health Issues* 21, no. 3 (2011): 187-190. doi: 10.1016/j.whi.2011.02.007.

Major-Kincade, Terri, and Kiley Hanish, *Challenging the Superwoman Mentality in the Black Community after Pregnancy and Infant Loss* (webinar). Return to Zero: H.O.P.E., June 24, 2020. RTZHope.org/webinar.

McCabe-Beane, Jennifer E., et al., "The Identification of Severity Ranges for the Edinburgh Postnatal Depression Scale," *Journal of Reproductive and Infant Psychology* 34, no. 3 (2014): 293–303. doi: 10.1080/02646838.2016.1141346.

McFarlane, Nichia, "U.S. Maternal Mortality Points to Institutional Racism. Is Philanthropy Listening to Black Women?" National Committee for Responsive Philanthropy, April 23, 2019. NCRP.org/2019/04/u-s-maternal-mortality -points-to-institutional-racism-is-philanthropy-listening-to-black-women.html.

Meyer, Birdie Gunyon, Daniel Singley, Kendra Flores-Carter, and Alison Reminick, "Perinatal Mood Disorders: Components of Care," Postpartum Support Inter- national's Two-Day Certificate of Completion Program, December 11–12, 2019, San Diego, CA.

Miller, William R., and Stephen Rollnick. *Motivational Interviewing: Helping People Change*. New York: Guilford Press, 2013.

Mongan, Marie F. *HypnoBirthing: The Mongan Method, A Natural Approach to Safer, Easier, More Comfortable Birthing*. London: Souvenir Press, 2016.

Motherly, "Motherly's 2019 State of Motherhood Survey Results," *Mother.ly*, December 30, 2019. Mother.ly/2019-state-of-motherhood-survey.

Nazish, Noma, "What Meghan Markle (and Other New Moms) Can Expect in the 'Fourth Trimester.'" *Forbes Magazine*, May 16, 2019, retrieved March 31, 2020, from Forbes.com/sites/nomanazish/2019/05/13/what-meghan-markle-and -other-new-moms-can-expect-in-the-fourth-trimester/.

O'Connor, Elizabeth, et al., "Primary Care Screening for and Treatment of Depression in Pregnant and Postpartum Women: Evidence Report and Systematic Review for the US Preventive Services Task Force," *JAMA* 315, no. 4 (2016): 388–406. doi: 10.1001/jama.2015.18948.

O'Connor, Elizabeth, et al., "Interventions to Prevent Perinatal Depression: Evidence Report and Systematic Review for the US Preventive Services Task Force," *JAMA* 321, no. 6 (2019): 588–601. doi: 10.1001/jama.2018.20865.

O'Hanlon, Bill. *Out of the Blue: Six Non-Medication Ways to Relieve Depression*. New York: W. W. Norton & Company, 2014.

O'Leary, Joann, "Subsequent Pregnancy: Healing to Attach after Perinatal Loss," *BMC Pregnancy and Childbirth* 15, Suppl. 1 (2015): A15. doi: 10.1186/1471 -2393-15-S1-A15.

O'Mahen, Heather, et al., "A Pilot Randomized Controlled Trial of Cognitive Behavioral Therapy for Perinatal Depression Adapted for Women with Low Incomes," *Depres- sion and Anxiety* 30, no. 7 (2013): 679–687. doi: 10.1002/da.22050.

Panahi, Faeze, and Mahbobeh Faramarzi, "The Effects of Mindfulness-based Cognitive Therapy on Depression and Anxiety in Women with Premenstrual Syndrome," *Depression Research and Treatment* 2016 (2016): 1–7. doi: 10.1155/2016/9816481.

Pearson, Rebecca M., et al., "The Normalisation of Disrupted Attentional Processing of Infant Distress in Depressed Pregnant Women Following Cognitive Behavioural Therapy," *Journal of Affective Disorders* 145, no. 2 (2013): 208–213. doi: 10.1016/j.jad.2012.07.033.

Pettman, Danelle, et al., "Effectiveness and Acceptability of Cognitive-Behavioural Therapy Based Interventions for Maternal Peripartum Depression: A Systematic Review, Meta-Analysis and Thematic Synthesis Protocol." *BMJ Open* 9, no. 12 (2019): e032659. doi: 10.1136/bmjopen-2019-032659.

Postpartum Support International, "Discussion Tool: Postpartum Support International (PSI)," accessed April 4, 2020. Postpartum.net/resources/discussion-tool/.

Reminick, Alison, "Pharmacologic Treatment of Mood Disorders in Pregnancy, Postpartum and Lactation," Postpartum Support International's 2-Day Certificate of Completion Program, December 12, 2019, San Diego, CA.

Reminick, Alison (Director, UCSD Women's Reproductive Mental Health Program). Personal communication with author, San Diego, CA, July 2020.

Saxbe, Darby E., et al., "High Paternal Testosterone May Protect against Postpartum Depressive Symptoms in Fathers, but Confer Risk to Mothers and Children," *Hormones and Behavior* 95 (2017): 103–112. doi: 10.1016/j.yhbeh.2017.07.014.

Schwartz, Jeffrey M., and Beverly Beyette. *Brain Lock: Free Yourself from Obsessive-Compulsive Behavior: A Four-Step Self-Treatment Method to Change Your Brain Chemistry*. New York: Harper Perennial, 2016.

Screening for Perinatal Depression—American College of Obstetricians and Gynecologists (ACOG), October 29, 2016. Retrieved on March 30, 2020, from ACOG.org/Clinical/Clinical-Guidance/Committee-Opinion/Articles/2018/11/Screening-for-Perinatal-Depression.

Sharma, Verinder, and Dwight Mazmanian, "The DSM-5 Peripartum Specifier: Prospects and Pitfalls," *Archives of Women's Mental Health* 17 (2014): 171–173. doi: 10.1007/s00737-013-0406-3.

Shulman, Barbara, et al., "Feasibility of a Mindfulness-based Cognitive Therapy Group Intervention as an Adjunctive Treatment for Postpartum Depression and Anxiety," *Journal of Affective Disorders* 235 (2018): 61–67. doi: 10.1016/j.jad.2017.12.065.

Sidebottom, Abbey, et al., "Perinatal Depression Screening Practices in a Large Health System: Identifying Current State and Assessing Opportunities to Provide More Equitable Care," *Archives of Women's Mental Health*, published online May 5, 2020, ahead of print. doi: 10.1007/s00737-020-01035-x.

Singley, D. B., and L. M. Edwards, "Men's Perinatal Mental Health in the Transition to Fatherhood," *Professional Psychology: Research and Practice* 46, no. 5 (2015), 309–316. doi: 10.1037/pro0000032.

Sockol, Laura E. "A Systematic Review of the Efficacy of Cognitive Behavioral Therapy for Treating and Preventing Perinatal Depression," *Journal of Affective Disorders* 177 (2015): 7–21. doi: 10.1016/j.jad.2015.01.052.

Stuart, Scott, and Michael D. Robertson. *Interpersonal Psychotherapy: A Clinician's Guide*. London: Hodder Arnold, 2012.

Tandoc, Edson C., Jr., Patrick Ferrucci, and Margaret Duffy, "Facebook Use, Envy, and Depression among College Students: Is Facebooking Depressing?," *Computers in Human Behavior* 43 (2015): 139–146. doi: 10.1016/j.chb.2014.10.053.

US Preventive Services Task Force, et al., "Interventions to Prevent Perinatal Depression: US Preventive Services Task Force Recommendation Statement," *JAMA* 321, no. 6 (2019): 580–587. doi: 10.1001/jama.2019.0007.

Uvnas-Moberg, Kerstin, and Kathleen Kendall-Tackett, "The Mystery of D-MER: What Can Hormonal Research Tell Us about Dysphoric Milk-Ejection Reflex?" *Clinical Lactation* 9, no. 1 (2018): 23–29. doi: 10.1891/2158-0782.9.1.23.

Viguera, Adele C., et al., "Risk of Recurrence in Women with Bipolar Disorder during Pregnancy: Prospective Study of Mood Stabilizer Discontinuation," *The American Journal of Psychiatry* 164, no. 12 (2007): 1817–1824; quiz 1923. doi: 10.1176/appi.ajp.2007.06101639.

Wisner, Katherine L., et al., "Onset Timing, Thoughts of Self-Harm, and Diagnoses in Postpartum Women with Screen-Positive Findings," *JAMA Psychiatry* 70, no. 5 (2013): 490–498.

Yonkers, Kimberly A., et al., "The Management of Depression during Pregnancy: A Report from the American Psychiatric Association and the American College of Obstetricians and Gynecologists," *General Hospital Psychiatry* 31 (2009): 403–413.

INDEX

ACKNOWLEDGMENTS

To my husband. I couldn't imagine adding one more thing on our plates. Yet, I said, hey, I'm writing a book in my "free time." Then a pandemic hit and the schools closed. Thank you for all the encouragement when I couldn't imagine another late night, early morning, or week without days off from writing.

To all who survived parenting and working from home in the age of COVID. In solidarity.

To the girls who made me a mother. You are forever my hearts, outside my body. I'm so proud and lucky that you are each the best of us.

To Dr. Alison Reminick for sharing her knowledge of reproductive psychiatry. To Joe Freeman and Michelle Routhieaux of the San Diego Depression Bipolar Support Alliance (DBSA) for the generous use of the Mood State Pyramid. To Suzanne Whittemore, Colleen Auth, and Dr. Raymond Fidaleo of the Sharp Mesa Vista Hospital Cognitive Therapy Intensive Outpatient Program, where I first learned GRAPES.

To PSI, PHA, MGH Women's Mental Health, the Postpartum Stress Center, and all my perinatal mental health colleagues. I have learned so much from you and hope I never stop.

ABOUT THE AUTHOR

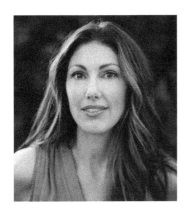

Abigail Burd, LCSW, PMH-C, is a perinatal mental health specialist in San Diego, California, at Burd Psychotherapy. She is a licensed clinical social worker and certified in perinatal mental health (psychotherapy) by Postpartum Support International. Abby is passionate about the postpartum stage and is humbled by the privilege of becoming a parent to two daughters. Abby is a member of the Postpartum Health Alliance and has served on its executive board. In 2019, she started an online fourth trimester school and launched the courses "Relationships After Baby" and "Prevent Postpartum Depression," which are based on the evidence-based strategies of cognitive behavioral therapy (CBT) and interpersonal psychotherapy (IPT). Burd is a board-certified diplomate (BCD) in clinical social work. Visit BurdTherapy.com to learn more about the author, follow @burdtherapy on Instagram/Twitter, or check out "Burd Psychotherapy and Education" on Facebook.

CPSIA information can be obtained
at www.ICGtesting.com
Printed in the USA
JSHW011916310721
17249JS00001B/1